PAINT YOUR STRESS AWAY

Hanaa F. Al-Wardi, MA, MFA

PAINT YOUR
STRESS AWAY

PAINT YOUR STRESS AWAY

THE BOOK ON ART
AS A THERAPEUTIC TOOL

Hanaa F. Al-Wardi, MA, MFA

www.hagallery.com

www.paintyourstressaway.com

Book Cover Art by Hanaa F. Al-Wardi
"Dust Storm" Acrylic on Canvas

Book Cover Design by Robert Allen

Book Formatting by Hani Jouni

Published by
MOCAA Publishing
225 West Main Street
Alhambra, CA 91801
USA

Printed in the United States of America.
ISBN 978-0-9864020-0-5

CONTENTS

TABLE OF CONTENTS, CONTINUED

FOREWORD

Are you stressed out? Do you want to live a stress-free life? If you are like most people, if you are a stressed-out professional or an overwhelmed parent, if you are always under financial pressure or always trying to meet deadlines, you can benefit from this book.

This book will teach you how to control and manage your stress using various artistic means and art therapy.

Paint Your Stress Away addresses a wide variety of stress related symptoms and suggests methods to control stress successfully through art before stress becomes a chronic and permanent condition. This book is practical, simple and easy to follow and is recommended to all readers who live under stressful conditions at home, at work, or in other areas of their lives. It is full of hints, techniques, guided imagery, and online video resources. The author also includes a list of personal stress reduction tips to incorporate on a daily basis throughout the book. This book demonstrates how to use art as a medium to transfer stress, anger, sorrow and frustration from your mind to your hand to a piece of paper or canvas. It is truly a cleansing process for your body and mind.

There is nothing better in life than to live with full control of your health and mood and experience relaxation, tranquility, and harmony. Reading this book will help guide you to the path of ownership of your mental and physical health. Use this book as a companion to improve your wellbeing and health. Once you have read it, go back and read it again to implement the techniques fully.

Just remember that there is nothing more important than maintaining your hope, improving your health, and experiencing mental peace and clarity. The result?

Less stress, increased happiness and a great sense of accomplishment!

I wish you great success on your artistic journey to health.

Raymond Aaron

NY Times Best Selling Author

INTRODUCTION

Let's face it: everybody is under some kind of stress, whether it is bad stress or good stress. Bad stress is very harmful if you don't control it and modify its destructive negative energy. Bad stress can harm your physical and mental health.

Good stresses are actually your passion and drive to do certain things that you love. When you do something you love, you are actually benefitting your health. Many studies reveal that the people who love what they do usually improve their mental strength and cognitive ability in their later years and they look more youthful and live much longer.

Your passion to do the things you love is a gift, so guard it and cherish every moment while doing it. Not many people are privileged and blessed to be in this situation.

There is nothing better than doing something you love. It is very energizing and exciting.

Paint Your Stress Away is my first book. It is a toolkit for life, offering many tips on how to incorporate art into your daily life to reduce stress, reduce pain, and uplift your soul and body. Art therapy can be used by everyone. You do not have to be a professional artist to reap its benefits.

As I researched the connection between art and health, I began to connect memories, personal stories and life experiences. The more I wrote about the art/mind/body connection, the more ideas started forming. This book was born of a truly amazing process of self-reflection and research and has opened the floodgates of my knowledge and my real life experiences as an artist.

I am a full time artist and a full time manager of my husband's neurology clinic. I feel that I am in a very unique position between my two worlds. At the clinic, patients seek treatment for a wide variety of serious illnesses from strokes to brain tumors, Parkinson's disease and Alzheimer's. A majority of patients seek treatment for migraines, tension headaches, anxiety and panic attacks, muscle tension, depression, ADHD, fibromyalgia and all other kinds of chronic aches and pains.

Usually, the patients check in with me before consulting with the doctor. I hear about their problems, stories of their stress and tense environments, and past traumatic experiences. My observation is that most patients experience high levels of bad stress.

Stress comes in so many forms, including high-pressure jobs, a demanding boss, an abusive spouse, children, long commutes, trauma, tests, illness, and so much more.

My career as a multimedia studio artist allows me to observe patients at the clinic through the lens of my art. As an artist, I am very visual and descriptive and appreciate all the details and the little things in life. I deal with a wide variety of mediums when I decide to create art. I keep my mind open to all possibilities and options. The sky is the limit when I create. I do not put obstacles or boundaries in my way. The ideas, materials, solutions and the stories I use are variable and endless. One story leads to another and goes on and on.

My experience in writing this book has led me to believe that I have so much to offer through a combination of artistic creation, inspiration, problem solving, and stress reduction. Art therapy combines all of this.

I hope you, the reader, will benefit from the approaches, methods, media and suggestions described as art therapy in this book. I hope that this book will give you the knowledge and tools to alleviate your stress and improve other various illnesses and conditions. Take your time to read and fully absorb the information in this book.

Check out the resources and web links and reap the full benefit of art therapy. Relax and enjoy!

Hanaa F. Al-Wardi

ACKNOWLEDGMENTS

To all the people who helped me shape this book and have made my life and work as bright and spectacular as it is today, thank you.

To my husband Dhia and my son Samir thank you for your brilliant ideas and continuous support.

And to my daughter Ban, thank you for your never ending support, thank you for believing in me, cheering me on and encouraging me throughout writing this book.

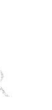

PAINT YOUR
STRESS AWAY

ARTIST/AUTHOR
STATEMENT

Hanaa F. Al-Wardi is an Iraqi-born multimedia studio artist based in Southern California. She received her Master's Degree in Medical Microbiology from California State University, Long Beach, and a Master's Degree in Fine Arts from the Claremont Graduate School in Claremont. She is the founder of the Museum of Contemporary Arab Art (MOCAA) based in Alhambra, California. MOCAA was founded in 2000 as a non-profit private organization to exhibit her work and host highly accomplished artists from around the Arab world. The author exhibits her work nationally and internationally and has participated in numerous discussions and television panels on her artwork. Her artwork features political issues, personal stories, and environmental concerns. A short list of her most prominent exhibits include:

- Operation Desert Slaughter
- Iraq Is Brain Dead
- Soft Target
- Collateral Damage
- Exposed

- Letters To The President
- Acid Rain
- Reaction
- Home
- Destiny
- Dismantling

For a closer look of **Hanaa Al-Wardi's** art, please visit her website: www.hagallery.com

This book was written for the many people who live with stress and many other health conditions that may benefit from art therapy. This book is meant to share how art can be used to enhance mental and physical wellbeing while also expressing ideas and thoughts on issues that are dear to the artist's heart and mind.

NOTE TO THE READER/DISCLAIMER

The information provided in this book is designed to provide helpful information on the subjects discussed. This book is not meant to be used, nor should it be used, to diagnose or treat any medical or psychological condition. For diagnosis or treatment of any medical or psychological problem, consult your own physician. The publisher and author are not responsible for any specific health or allergy needs that may require medical supervision and are not liable for any damages or negative consequences from any treatment, action, application or preparation, to any person reading or following the information in this book. References, including photos and artistic images, are provided for informational and demonstration purposes only. Use of these photos and images are not intended for commercial use. They do not constitute an endorsement of any website or other source. Readers should be aware that the websites and alternate contact information listed in this book may change.

PAINT YOUR
STRESS AWAY

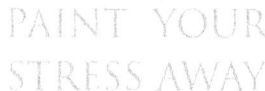

CHAPTER 1

THE
MANY SHADES
OF RELAXATION
METHODS

T he effects of stress on individuals are variable; it can manifest itself as migraine headaches, backaches, ADHD, depression, anxiety, eating disorders and many other health conditions. Different people have different coping mechanisms to deal with stress and its consequences. More and more people are beginning to accept and understand alternative solutions for many of their illnesses and to overcome their stress outside of mainstream medicine.

1

Perhaps this realization came from the numerous side effects of prescription medicines. People are finding relief for their symptoms and pain through alternative treatments. Art therapy is one such therapy.

The process of creating art has been shown to aid in many conditions, including heart disease, influenza, and even cancer. The emotional devastation and fallout from illness can be eased through creative methods. Many studies show that patients engaged in art therapy have better vital signs and sleep much better too.

Creative activities and mindful art are very important to lower the stress level on the body and the immune system. It can help improve your wellbeing and performance, boost your productivity at work, and even improve your interactions with your clients, co-workers and your family members. I have

The emotional devastation and fallout from illness can be eased through creative methods. Many studies show that patients engaged in art therapy have better vital signs and sleep much better too.

found that abstract art is the best method; just use paint and use your hands, applying, removing, and adding anything you want, anything you wish: who cares? Just express yourself! Splattering paint all over will really make you feel good. It's like child's play: all fun, no worries, spontaneous, intuitive and happy. It doesn't have to be paint; creativity can be expressed through flower arranging, dancing, cooking, gardening, or rearranging the furniture. Any and all of the above activities will help your brain cope with stress. Collage art also works very well to get to the bottom of a stressful situation, and for finding creative ways to solve your stressful situation.

Art can be used to help people communicate, overcome stress and explore different aspects of their own personality. In psychology, the use of artistic methods to treat psychological disorders and enhance mental health is known as art therapy.

Art therapy integrates psychotherapeutic techniques with the creative process to improve mental health and wellbeing. The American Art Therapy Association describes art therapy as "a mental health profession that uses the creative process of art making to improve and enhance the physical, mental and emotional wellbeing of individuals of all ages. It is based on their belief that the creative process involved in artistic self-expression helps people to resolve conflicts and problems, develop interpersonal , manage behavior, decrease stress, increase self-esteem and self-awareness and achieve insights."

Just looking at pictures of a beautiful serene landscape in the hospital or home has been shown to reduce the need for narcotics and speed up recovery time. Another study showed that some cancer patients respond well to art therapy programs because it gives them an identity outside of their diagnosis. Emotional stress can be relieved, and even some physical symptoms can be diminished. Engaging in drawing and painting activities will definitely relax you tremendously; it gets your thoughts more focused on the art project and distracts you from your stressful situation.

Sketching and journaling to describe your inner feelings also helps a lot. When you are engaged in creative activities, it has a calming effect, reducing blood pressure dramatically, as shown in many clinical studies.

My family has an annual ritual every New Year's Eve. We all gather around the fireplace and write any or all of what is

Engaging in drawing and painting activities will definitely relax you tremendously; it gets your thoughts more focused on the art project and distracts you from your stressful situation.

bothering us, from health issues to bad experiences at work, bad friendships and many other negative things. At the end,

I collect all the papers and burn them in the fireplace and delete them from our memories. The feeling of doing it is wonderful, and we start fresh for the New Year. It is a very positive practice for you to use to cleanse your life of negative energy you might have collected throughout the year. It is a very exciting event for all members of my family and even our friends. It is really such a joyful, energetic and happy practice for all of us, and we look forward to it every year.

Other stress relief activities could be working with clay, gardening, arranging flowers, knitting, reading, playing music, digital art, dancing, eating dark chocolate, playing with pets, loud laughter, calling loved ones, gossiping and whispering, walking in the park, or yoga. Actually, the best stress relief activity is yawning and stretching.

Working with clay is an amazing experience, it is very soothing. Touching the clay, manipulating the clay, forming and caring for the object is an amazing feeling. You will totally forget your problems and stress. You feel very calm and accomplished and at the end, you are creating something. The process doesn't end here; you still have to care for the object and handle it with sensitivity until it is totally dry and then fire it. You trust the fire to take care of your object. The firing process raises anxiousness and feelings about the unpredictability of the outcome. If it survives the fire and your object comes out of the kiln intact, you still have to do more. You have to glaze it and dry again, and give it to the fire again, and wait patiently for the fire and the heat to cool down. Next, you open the door of the kiln and pray to God that the results are to your satisfaction and what you imagined it to be. This is a totally different level of experience.

Working with clay, is a life changing process. It will definitely make you more patient, more flexible and more accepting of failures, mistakes and disappointments. You become more trusting and accepting of harsh environments. Clay teaches you that hard work, obstacles and extreme heat will eventually

Working with clay is an amazing experience, it is very soothing. Touching the clay, manipulating the clay, forming and caring for the object is an amazing feeling.

produce the outcome you desire. It will polish your personality and temper your mood and will teach you that life is not an easy street, everything rosy, easy, and comfortable.

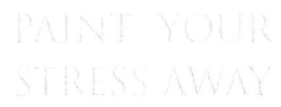

PHOTOS OF SELECTED CERAMIC ART BY HANAA AL-WARDI

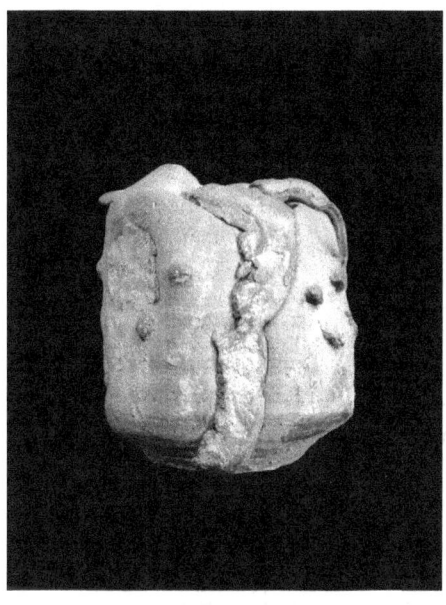

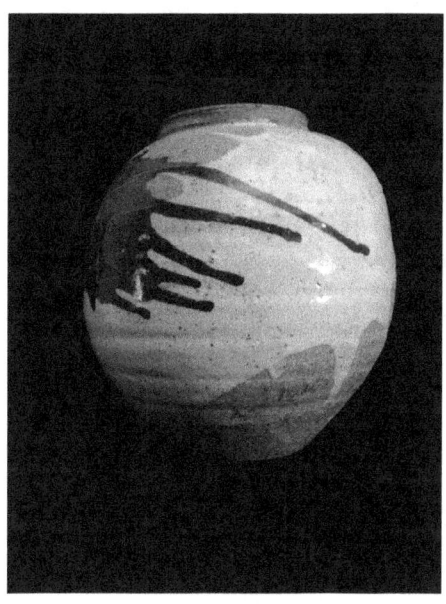

PHOTOS OF SELECTED CERAMIC ART BY HANAA AL-WARDI

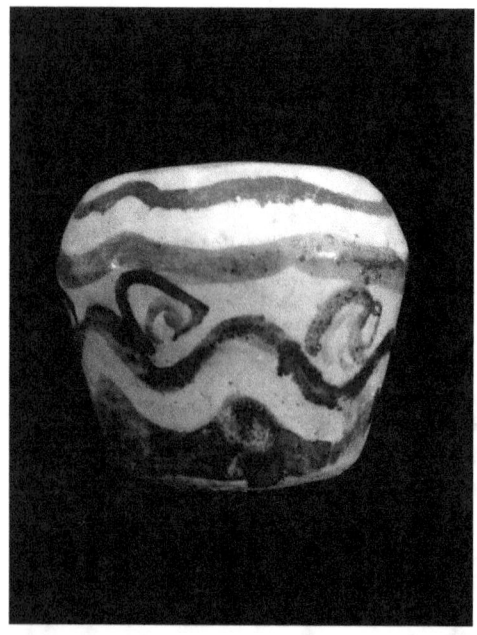

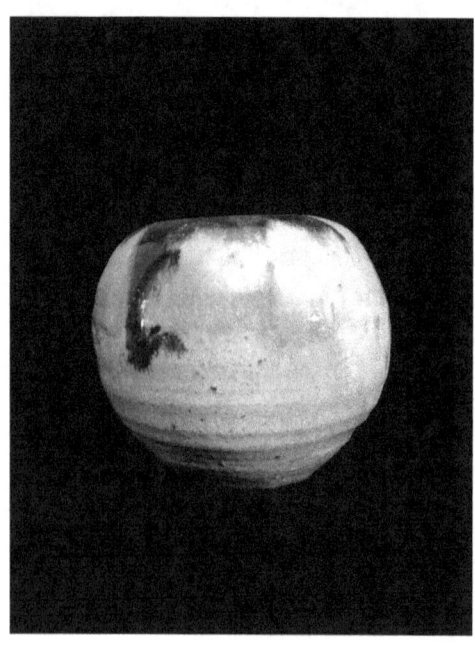

PHOTOS OF SELECTED CERAMIC ART BY HANAA AL-WARDI

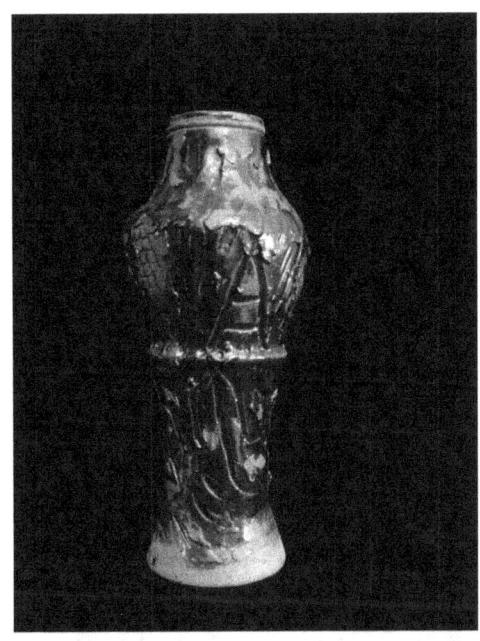

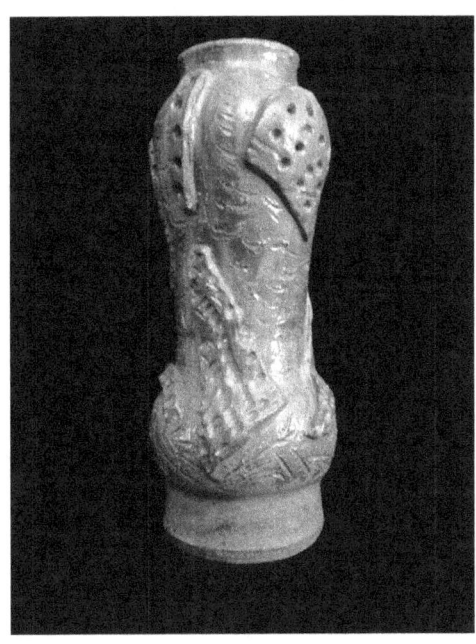

PHOTOS OF SELECTED CERAMIC ART BY HANAA AL-WARDI

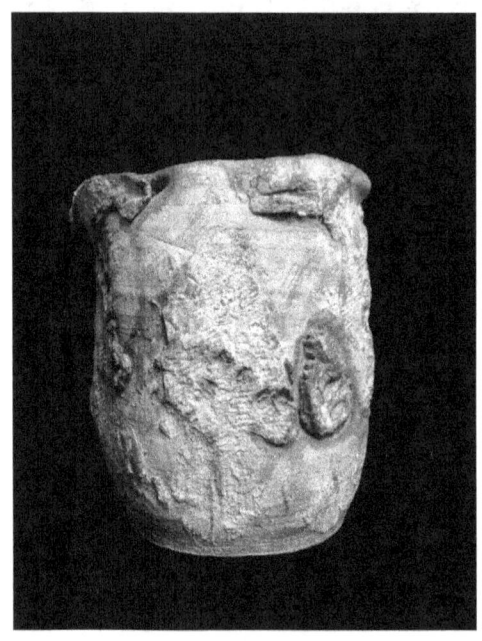

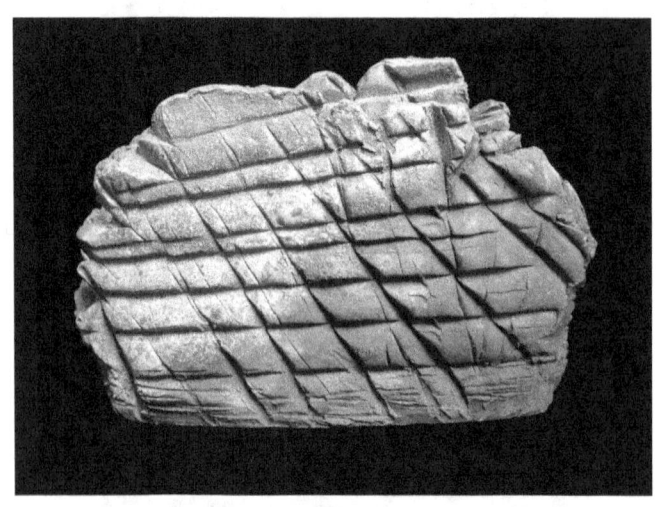

PHOTOS OF SELECTED CERAMIC ART BY HANAA AL-WARDI

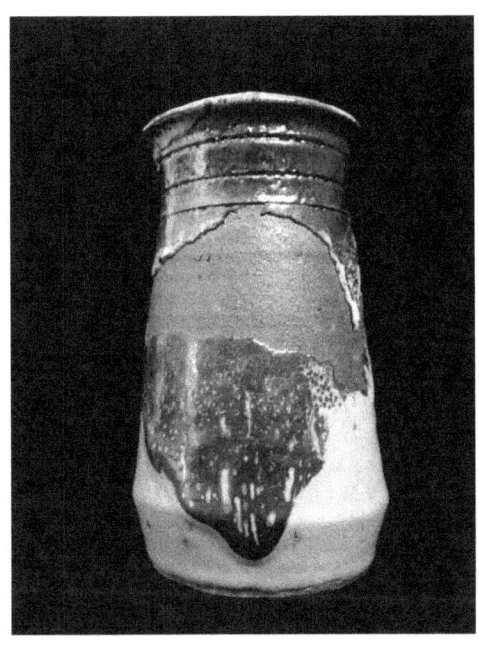

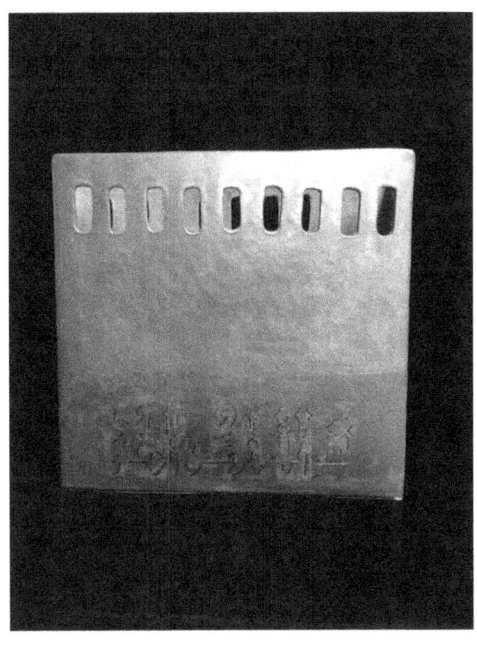

PHOTOS OF SELECTED CERAMIC ART BY HANAA AL-WARDI

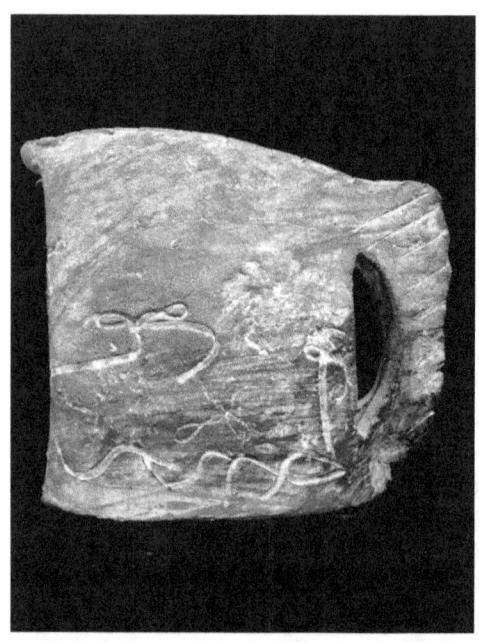

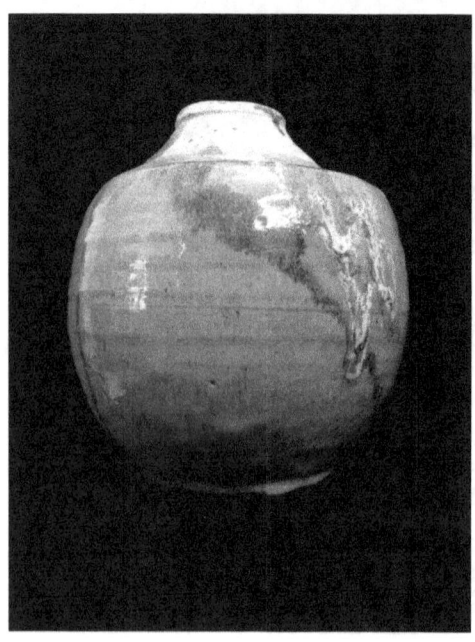

PHOTOS OF SELECTED CERAMIC ART BY HANAA AL-WARDI

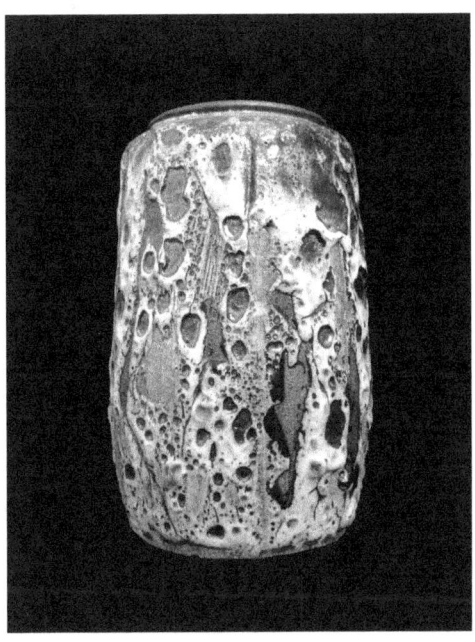

Years ago when my mother passed away, her death was unexpected and premature. I was struck by a monumental grief and never left home for several weeks. It was a tremendous shock to my entire family, and especially for me. I was living far away from her at that time. I used to be very protective and very close to her, and her death hit me very hard. I was crying continuously. I had no control of my tears, so I took solace with art and started knitting and knitting. I used to sit next to the fireplace, watching the flame and feeling the warmth of the fire knitting afghan blankets, brown, yellow and white in color, I still have it and use it. Few months of knitting, I felt much better. I ended up with numerous knitted Items. I produced so many sweaters, blankets, hats, shawls and wraps that it felt to me at that time as if I had transferred all my sorrow, grief and heartaches to all of the things I made. They are beautiful and full of care, love, tranquility and acceptance. That experience was very valuable to me, because I was alone dealing with the loss, but I had my mind and my subconscious mind to guide me through it. So the lesson from this story is, use your creative mind to guide you, to pull you through tragedy, sorrow and stress.

Calligraphic activities are very relaxing, especially when you are engaged in humming during the process. Humming increases the dopamine and serotonin level of your brain, both of the "feel-good hormones." Try it; you'll like it. Practice calligraphy with any color you want. Personally, I prefer black ink on white paper. It is very simple, and calming.

I write, create, and hum. (Please see "The Mindful Art of Thich Nhat Hanh" on YouTube, "Calligraphic Meditation," Nov. 4, 2011 and watch Oprah Winfrey interview with Thich Nhat Hanh, OWN Network, May 12, 2013).

There is calligraphy for meditation. The sutra "You are Nobody" is a poem written by Houzan Suzuki for one of his Japanese clients. It is a beautiful work of Japanese calligraphy. You can see this video on YouTube. This beautiful meditation calligraphy was published on September 20, 2009. There is also a Zen calligraphy demonstration by Harada Shodo Roshi, available on YouTube.

There are so many calligraphy meditation videos online. The music is unbelievable and soothing for anyone under stress (or no stress; it really doesn't matter). It just uplifts your mind and transforms you so you can inhabit a different state of mind. I suggest you try them all. Your life will be significantly enriched as a result.

If you watch "Meditate with Calligraphy" by Swami Anand Kul Bhushan in Delhi India, and watch him do his calligraphy and meditate, you will be amazed. The process is ancient. It has been a common practice in many religions from Buddhism to Islam to Christianity and others. They use calligraphy to convey their messages, and while doing it they were in a meditative state.

There is really a fantastic YouTube video, it's a must to watch, and its name is "Heart Sutra Meditation in calligraphy" by Ponte Ryuurui.

The "Calligraphy Moving Meditation Workshop with Pearl Weng Liang Huang" of Ru Yi Studio on YouTube is also wonderful. Pearl Huang's YouTube video is about Chinese brush calligraphy as the dance of life force and poetry in motion. It is a part of Tai Ji Gong Workshop at the City of Arcadia Community Center.

There is also a recitation of Al-Quran by a Muslim girl with an amazing voice, "Surat Al-Fajr," which means "The Dawn." Watch it on YouTube; when you listen to her, you will get the chills. Just close your eyes and listen. Even if you don't understand the words or the meanings, just hearing her voice will send you to a different level of consciousness.

The Whirling Dervishes are Turkish monks who turn in circles for hours to meditate and transcend to a different level of consciousness. By watching the process as an observer you will also achieve a meditative state and your blood pressure lowers down as if you are sedated. All of your stress and worries diminish, especially when you listen to their music. I personally experienced this process on a couple of occasions, once in Los Angeles, during a performance, and the second time when I traveled to Istanbul, Turkey. If you cannot see the activities in person or at a live show, I suggest you watch it on YouTube. Multiple links are included in the reference section as "The Sufi Whirling Dervishes of Istanbul." DVDs are also available for purchase. It is unbelievable. When I went to Istanbul a few years ago and listened to the music, I was mesmerized. Before my departure, I purchased the DVD from a store in the airport just before I boarded the plane. Sometimes I play it and watch it when I want to be totally relaxed and distract my attention from stressful situations. It will also help you to go to sleep easily.

I have measured my blood pressure before and after listening to the music, and usually my blood pressure drops by at least 10-15 points. When listening to the soothing or calming music, close your eyes and imagine beautiful scenes: waterfalls, the beach, or a field of flowers full of butterflies. That will definitely improve your mood and raise your positive energy.

I have measured my blood pressure before and after listening to the music, and usually my blood pressure drops by at least 10-15 points.

Art therapy can be used successfully as a means of communication. Drawing, painting, and other expressions of art are used to communicate conflict, struggles, and emotions. In this way, the art image helps the patient communicate with the therapist so that new insights are revealed. When this happens, they are much better equipped to resolve conflicts, solve problems, and create new perceptions that can lead to growth and healing.

While many people may be reluctant to engage in art therapy because they don't feel they have talent, anyone can use art therapy. The goal is not to create a masterpiece but to feel comfortable expressing oneself through artistic creation.

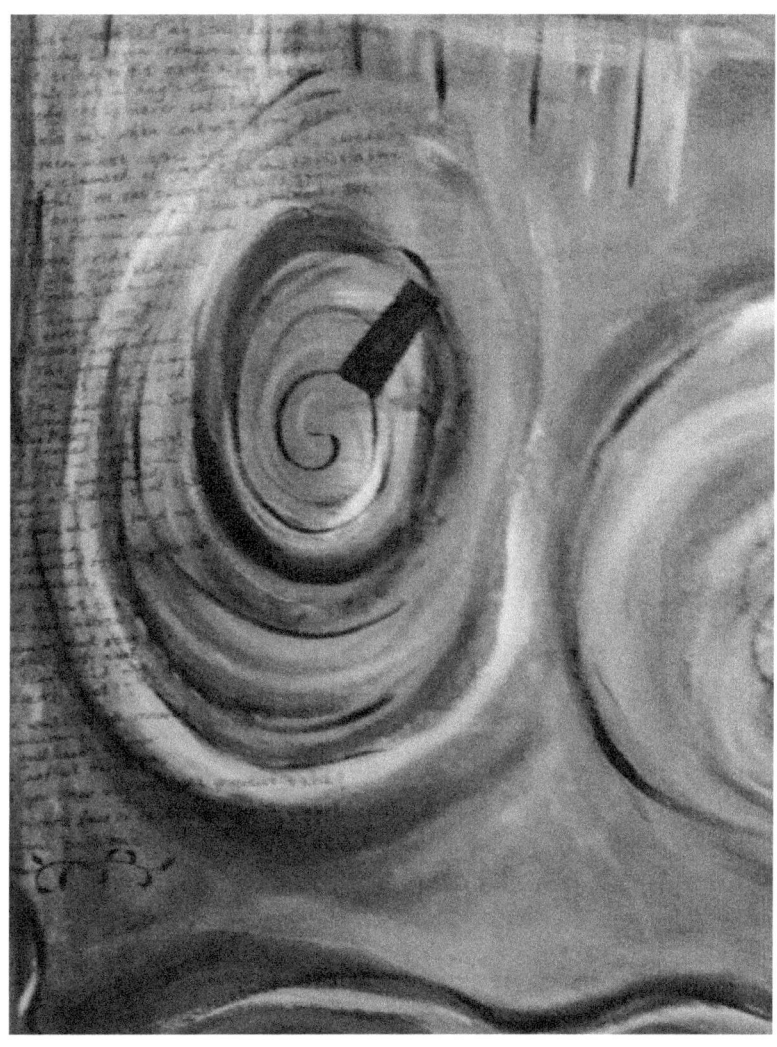

CHAPTER 2

THE
STRESS
TRAP

When you are under stress, you can be easily overwhelmed by feelings of tension, frustration, hostility, foggy thinking and anger. With these feelings, you feel down, like you are drowning or as if you are going through quick sand and there is no way out. When you are cornered, your body acts negatively and starts secreting the stress hormone "cortisol" which can harm you tremendously. Also, stress causes your blood pressure to rise and that is very harmful to your cardiovascular system and your heart. The stress hormone also harms your kidneys and your cognitive functions.

But by diverting your attention and focusing on something totally different, like artistic activities, the process by itself will pull you out of these stressful situations. Using art as a therapeutic and stress relief tool is a wonderful way for releasing stored up stress and anger, and to deal with other emotions and issues. The process will empower you through creativity and the expression of your inner feelings. Practicing art will enable and empower you to quickly shift your mood by releasing your anger and unhappiness almost instantaneously.

Practicing art will enable and empower you to quickly shift your mood by releasing your anger and unhappiness almost instantaneously.

You can practice art during your lunch break if you're working in a corporate environment or clinic (as I do). I do my relaxation practice during my lunch break. I listen to soft music, what I call "healing music." My favorite is Andrew Weil, M.D.'s "Sound Body Sound Mind," music for healing. I always play it as background music in the clinic, and I highly recommend it. It will help you in your journey to health and inner peace. I listen to it over and over during the day and especially when I take walks after long, demanding days at the clinic. It makes me feel refreshed and alert.

Another great stress relief method is art viewing or clipping pictures from magazines for a future art project. This approach usually changes my perspective on everything and deflates any stress I am feeling.

A few years ago, I went to a neck and spine specialist to check my neck after an injury. After he examined me, I said, "Please tell me how I can avoid future injury or damage." His answer was **"stop living."** So the moral of the story is that if you are living, you will experience life issues, health problems, losses, separations and other problems. You have to learn how to cope. I will show you methods in this book that work and give you the tools to help reduce/manage stress on daily basis.

Years ago, I went through remodeling my house. The process was so stressful and exhausting every step of the way. I was totally drained, tired, exhausted and desperate for the project to end. Then, I thought of using all the leftover house paint I had in my garage. I splattered all the colors on a very large piece of canvas. I used the left over plaster, sandpaper, wood and even nails and screws to produce texture, and poured coffee over the canvas to stain it. The end result was a smashing success; I still have it and I cherish it. That approach helped me cleanse my stress and disappointment. Needless to say, I started fresh and started enjoying my house and felt happy, and when I am happy, everybody in the family is happy.

So just be yourself, set yourself free, explore and have fun; it will affect your psychological wellbeing tremendously. When you engage in artistic activities and create, your spirit and mood will be uplifted. You will feel that you can deal with daily activities and daily stresses. It will also help everybody around you.

If you are living, you will experience life issues, health problems, losses, separations and other problems. You have to learn how to cope. I will show you methods in this book that work and give you the tools to help reduce/manage stress on daily basis.

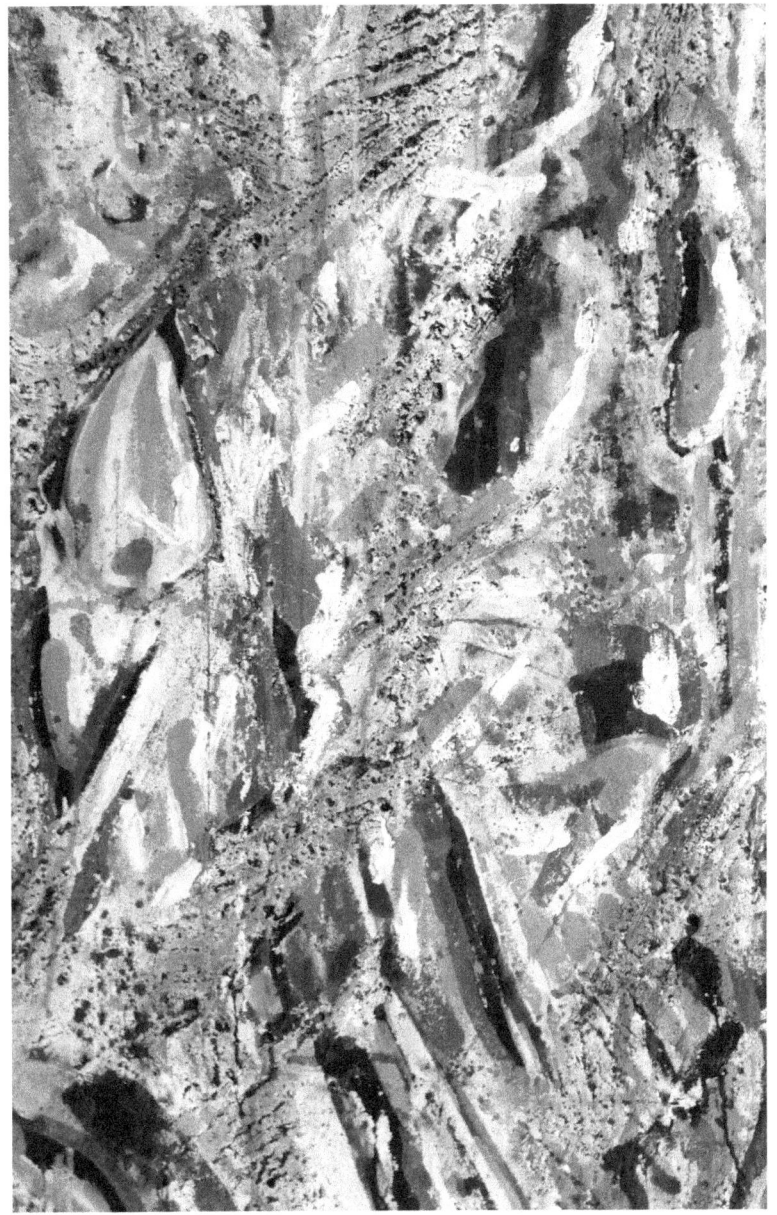

REMODELING, 1994 - Mixed Media

EXAMPLES OF ABSTRACT ART

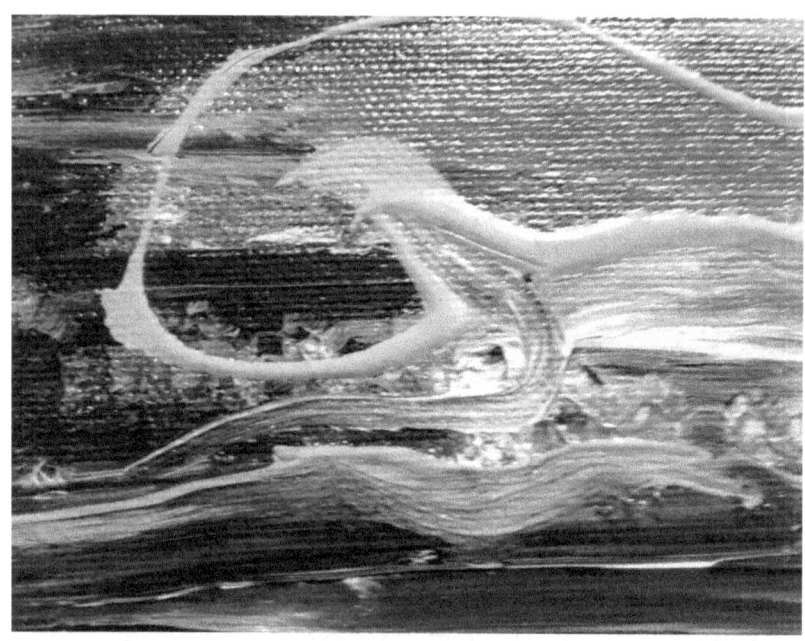

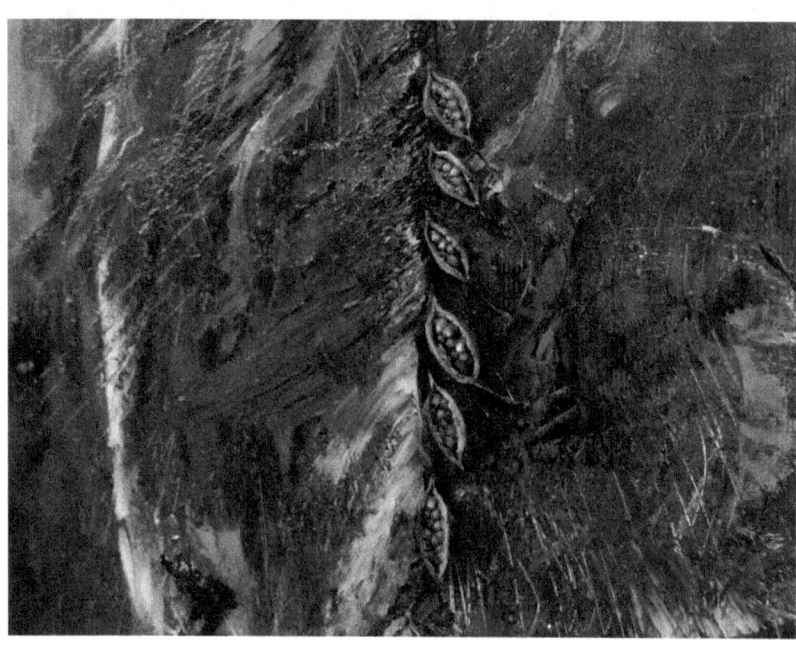

CHAPTER 3

DO-IT YOURSELF ART THERAPY

You don't have to be a professional artist or graduate art student to incorporate art therapy into your everyday life. Abstract art is really my favorite, and it is the easiest and surest method to change your mood. It will enable you to express your inner feelings easily and release your inner hostilities and feelings of helplessness.

The beauty of abstract art is that there are no restrictions or rules to follow; just freely express your emotions and inner thoughts, and who knows what will come? You could choose a piece of wood and glue any kind of object on it, or create symbols of your problems. It might lead you to solve your problems when you look at them from a different perspective. Actually, when you paint a subject or do a collage piece, you transfer your problem from your mind and body to the piece on the wall or on the table. You are removing the problem from your body as if it is a third-person (out of body experience), as if your problem is just an object that can be changed and manipulated, or even destroyed. I guarantee you if you adapt this approach to deal with your stress and problems you will be very successful in solving any problem you might face.

The beauty of abstract art is that there are no restrictions or rules to follow; just freely express your emotions and inner thoughts, and who knows what will come?

Even if you are not in the mood to paint or create something, or you think that you cannot paint or draw, think again; just close your eyes and think or imagine you are painting and creating. As an artist myself, sometimes I paint in my dreams. I just tell myself to paint before I sleep and tell my subconscious mind to remember it in the morning. You will be surprised and amazed what you come up with, it is really magical. You might think the actual process of artwork is different from the imaginative artwork I've just described, but really it is very effective and successful.

Even looking at pleasant artwork and nice scenery will lower your blood pressure and help to calm your pain. Also, if you listen to inspirational music while attempting to paint or do other creative activities, the music will definitely induce and activate the creative side of your brain.

When you paint a subject or do a collage piece, you transfer your problem from your mind and body to the piece on the wall or on the table.

Years ago, I had a very important experience that emphasized my belief in using art as a therapeutic tool and problem solving. I passed through very troublesome family confrontation and argument that I couldn't handle and I didn't want to invest my energy in dealing with it. My only refuge was art; I stayed awake all night long drawing, writing and painting. I totally immersed myself in what I was doing until the morning. In the morning, I was so tired, exhausted and dizzy that I did not pay attention to the results of my work. The next day after a long nap, I woke up fully rested. I went back and took a look at my work. I was so pleased and surprised that I entered the pieces in a local contest and I won. I also sold two pieces. I was so happy and relieved, and when I looked back at the family problem, to my surprise it wasn't that bad at all and it was easy to deal with. I realized that creativity cleansed my mind and purged the toxic thoughts that I was stuck with. It was a very good lesson for me, and I always remember it and use it.

I am an Iraqi born artist. I came to the United States in 1970 with my husband for further education. We lived the American dream and we had a wonderful life: great education, great profession, a beautiful house, and beautiful children until 1990 when the first Gulf War started.

I realized that creativity cleansed my mind and purged the toxic thoughts that I was stuck with. It was a very good lesson for me, and I always remember it and use it.

The bombing and the destruction that was inflicted on my homeland was awful. I was in total shock and sorrow. I was worried about my family, my extended family and dear friends. With the heavy bombing, communication was cut off totally. There was no way for me to know what happened to my brothers and sisters, nieces and nephews. I imagined that all of them had been killed, the bombing was so ferocious; in my mind, nobody could survive it.

I was glued to the TV and the radio to hear what was going on. I was frightened and scared of the unknown. I cried every time I imagined one of my siblings under the rubble, dead. I used to go to the Red Cross office and report the names of

There was no way for me to know what happened to my brothers and sisters, nieces and nephews. I imagined that all of them had been killed, the bombing was so ferocious; in my mind, nobody could survive it.

my siblings and family so they could track them and give me some news. I thought maybe they had escaped the bombs or became refugees somewhere in the desert.

I had no experience whatsoever with violent death or displacement. While I was writing the notes on a small postcard at the Red Cross, I was crying so badly that I couldn't breath. I was comforted by the staff and assured me that they would get me some news about my relatives. These were the saddest days of my life, because I was totally in the dark.

During that dark period, I kept myself busy with painting and expressing my deep sad feelings. I was writing a lot on the paintings; they were like a documentation of the war day by day, hour by hour. By the end of the war, I had finished six paintings, 4' x 6' each, depicting each period of the war. I also made a ceramic mural 5'x25'. I also collected letters from friends and family members and superimposed their faces on the letters, all in black and white, 24" x 36" each.

To my surprise, the act of painting was of great help to me, and I created a very important body of work to depict the war. I called that body of work *"Collateral Damage."* It was covered by ABC, NBC, BBC and CNN. For a closer look go to: www.hagallery.com.

I exhibited my work for two months, and then I made posters and postcards of each painting and was exhibited nationally and internationally. The exhibit ended up in the Museum of Contemporary Art in Baghdad. It was on display until the second war in 2003. The museum was looted and my art work was destroyed.

The exhibit ended up in the Museum of Contemporary Art in Baghdad. It was on display until the second war in 2003. The museum was looted and my art work was destroyed.

A few months went by and I received a message from my brother through NBC. He assured me that all my family members were okay and alive.

Without my expression through my art, my sadness, anxiety and worries would have taken over my life and my mental health. Art helped me even more. I sold the reprints of my work on posters and postcards. I raised funds to buy medicine, toys and teddy bears for the children of Iraq. Also, I received a huge donation of toys and teddy bears form well-wishers, kind people and pharmaceutical companies. Eventually, I went to Iraq with a nurse friend and delivered all the toys, the medicine and the teddy bears to the children myself. The experience was tremendous, very enriching and satisfying, and put closure on those very sad feelings I had experienced during the war. So when I say to use art as a therapeutic tool, I really speak from personal experience.

A few years after the war, the focus of the news became on the devastation of the environment in Iraq. The effect of the bombing became more obvious for the ordinary person. I lost many friends to cancer, others to ALS, and there were numerous deformities in the newly born babies of friends. The soil, water, and air all were contaminated. People started buying food from outside the country and even importing drinking water from outside.

I lost many friends to cancer, others to ALS, and there were numerous deformities in the newly born babies of friends.

My way of dealing with the horrible aftermath was to start a new body of work to expose the facts on the ground. I used metal, coins, chemicals and metal pipes to express my feelings and my thoughts on the destruction of the environment. I let the chemicals produce the art subjects, and each one depicted a different stage of destruction, contamination, oil spills and greed. I used cassette tapes, slides and satellite photos. That exhibit, titled *"Exposed,"* totaled thirteen pieces of different sizes. To see more go to: *www.hagallery.com.*

Years later, my feelings calmed down and I went back to my usual love of nature, the environment, colors and texture. I worked on a new body of work, called *"Color Melody."* It was full of colors, joy, hope and happiness. For a closer look at my work, please visit www.hagallery.com.

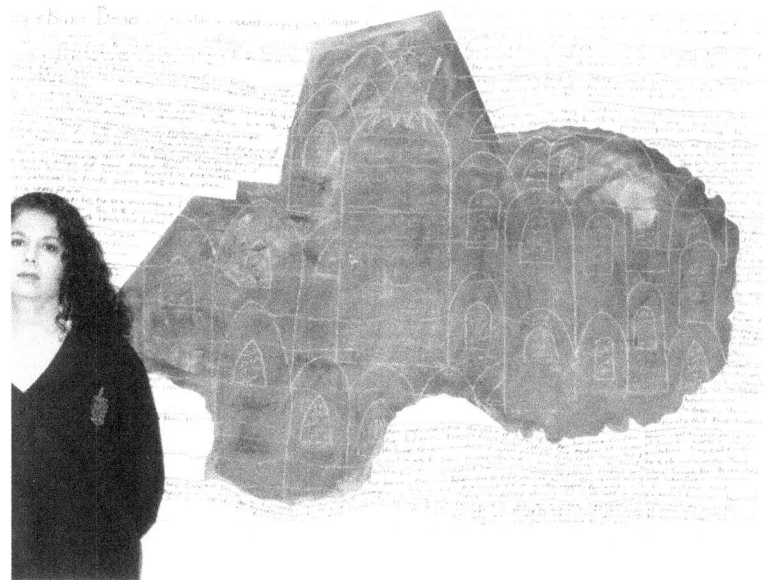

IRAQ IS BRAIN DEAD - 1992

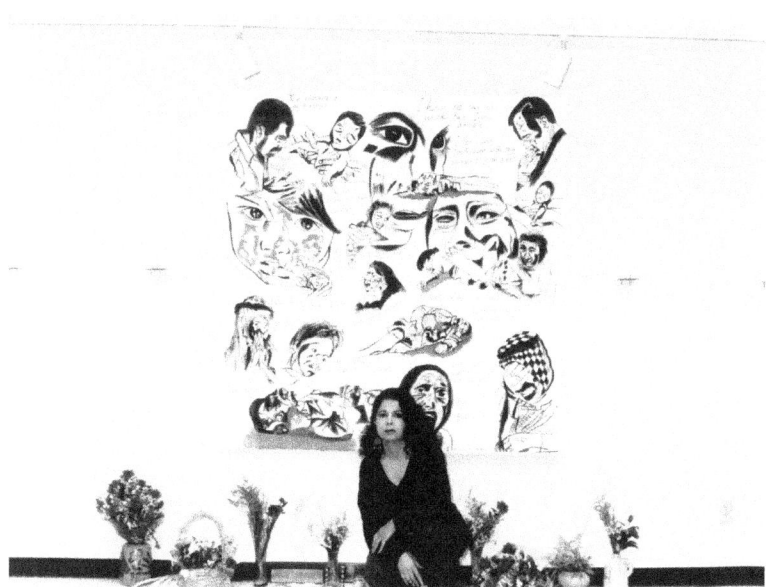

VICTORY - 1992

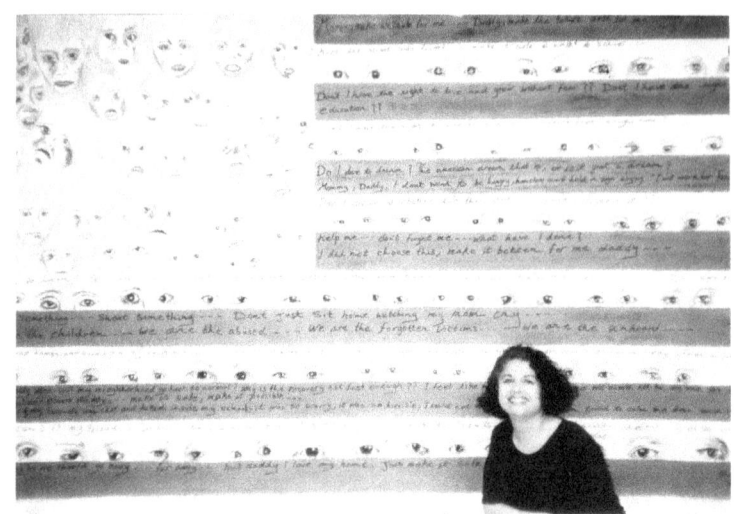

VOICES OF THE UNHEARD - 1992

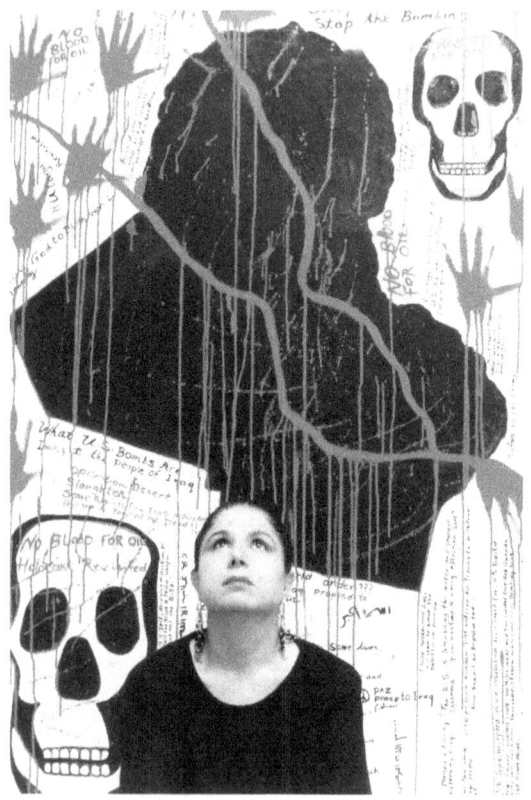

OPERATION DESERT SLAUGHTER - 1992

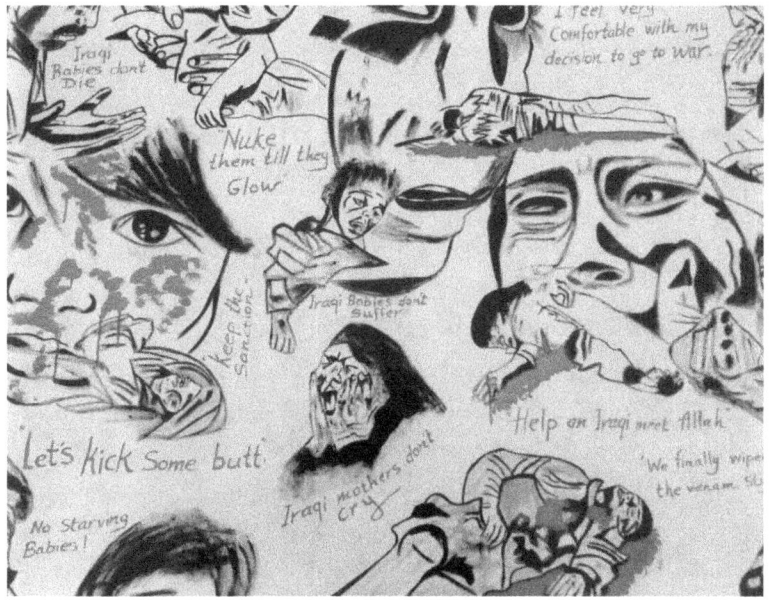

VICTORY - 1992

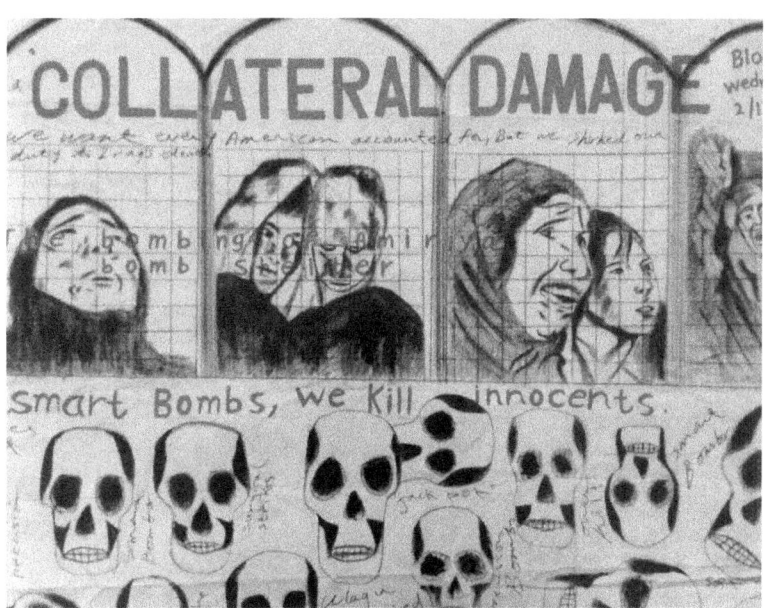

COLLATERAL DAMAGE - 1992

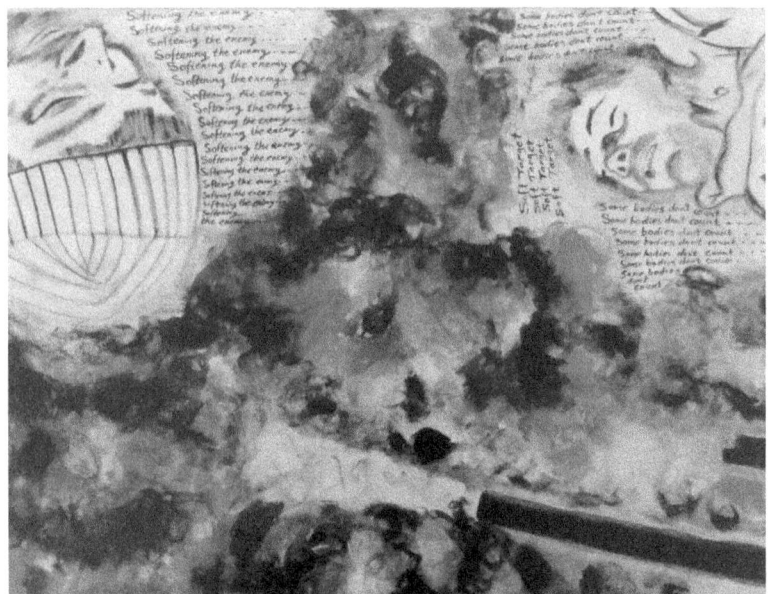

SOFT TARGET - 1992

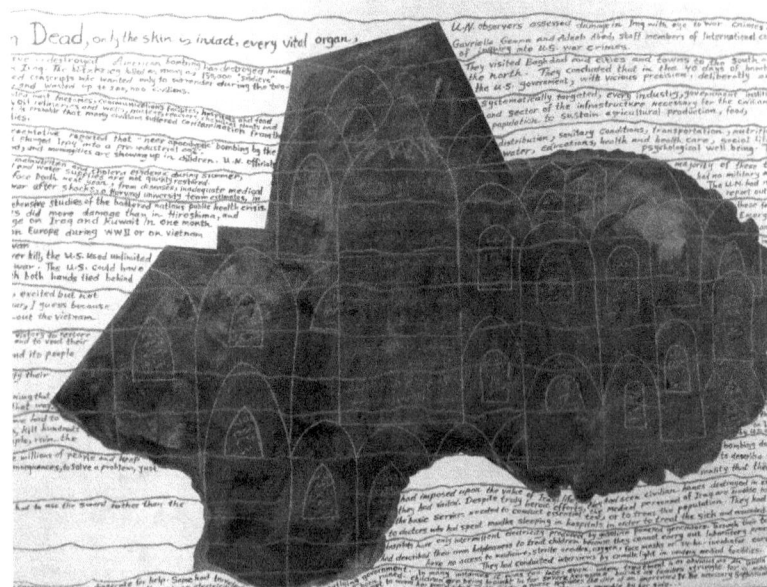

IRAQ IS BRAIN DEAD - 1992

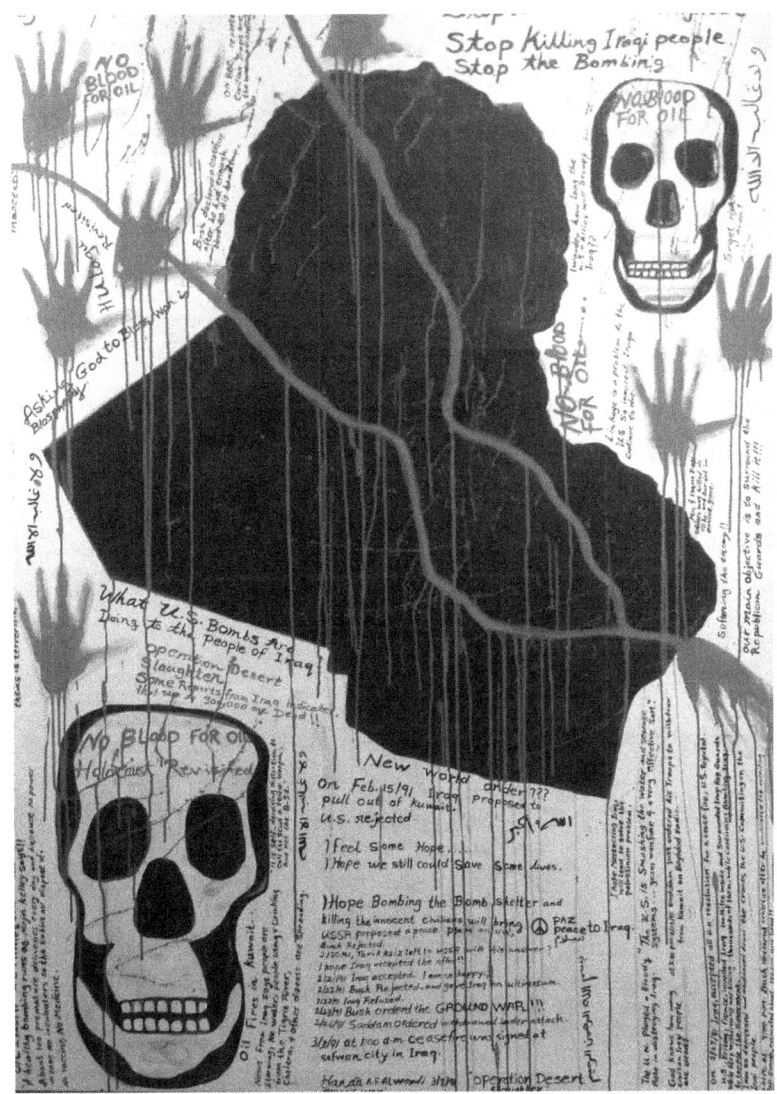

OPERATION DESERT SLAUGHTER - 1992

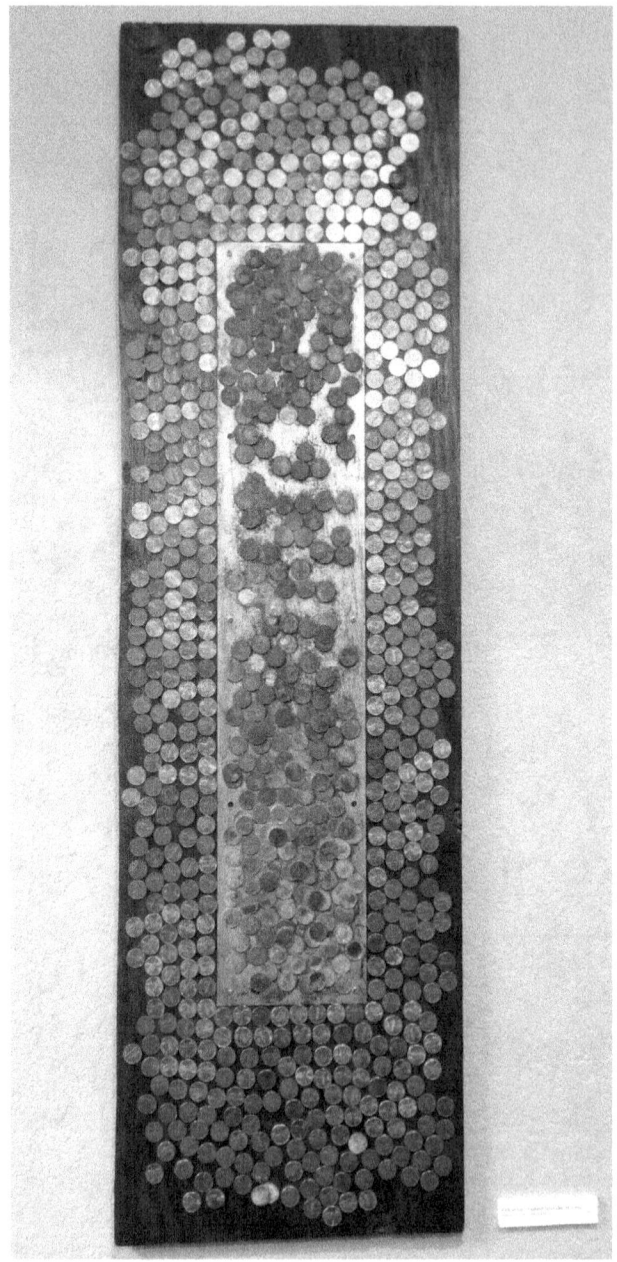

EXPENSIVE OIL - CHEAP MONARCHY - 1996

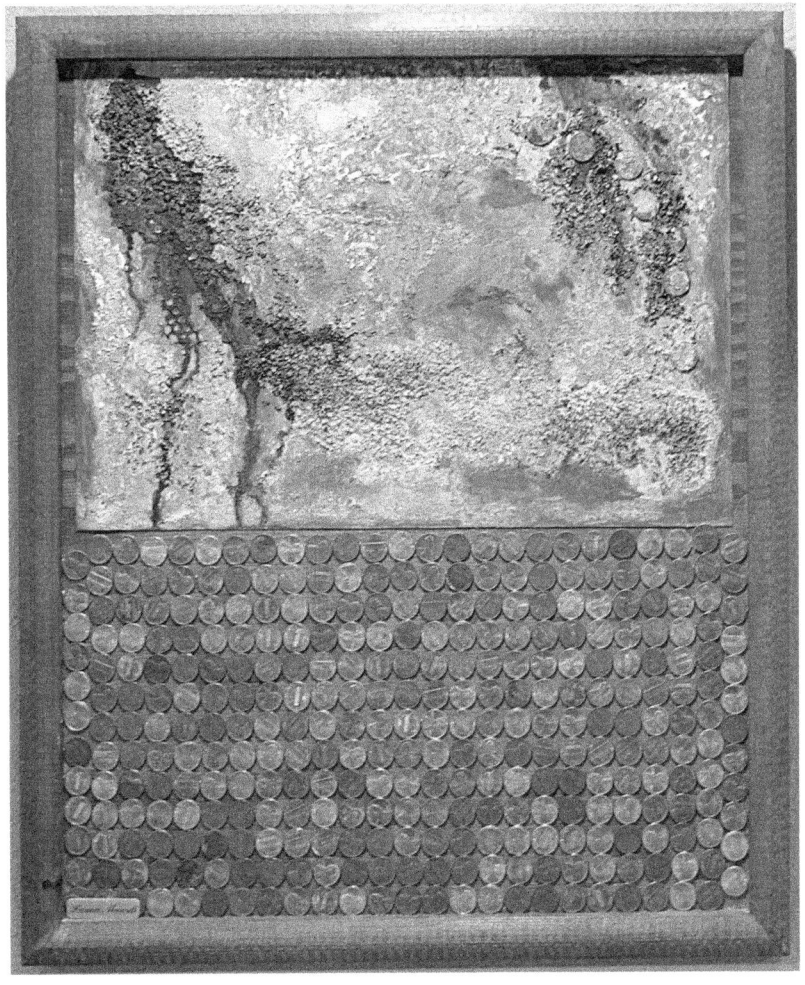

OIL SPILLS AND GREED - 1996

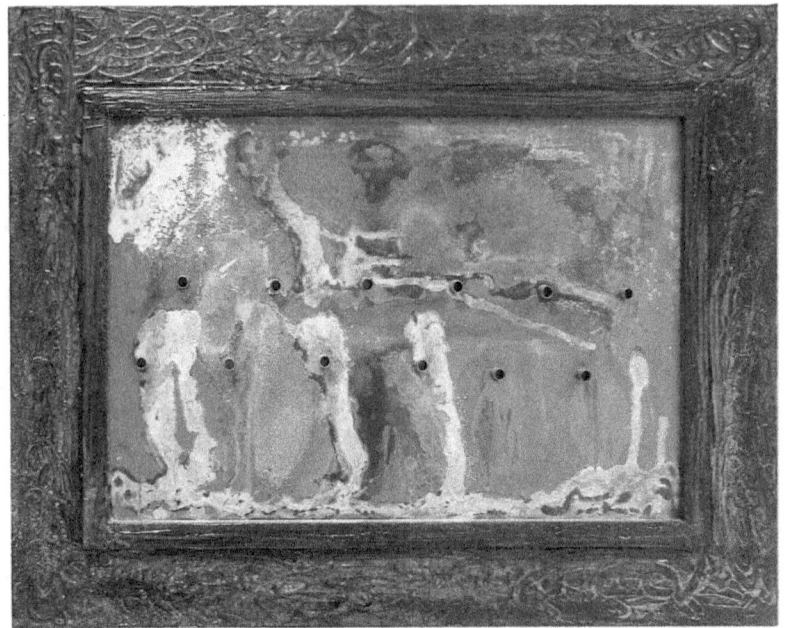

DISMANTLING - 1996

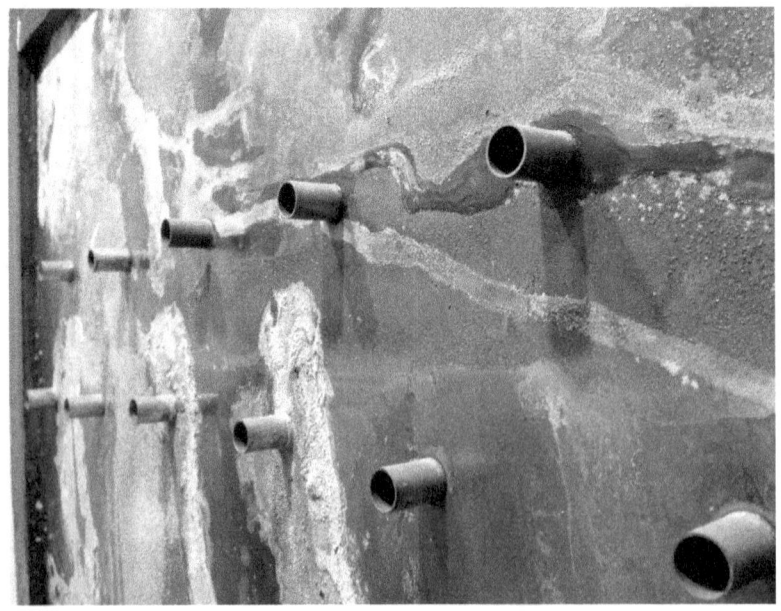

DISMANTLING - (close-up) 1996

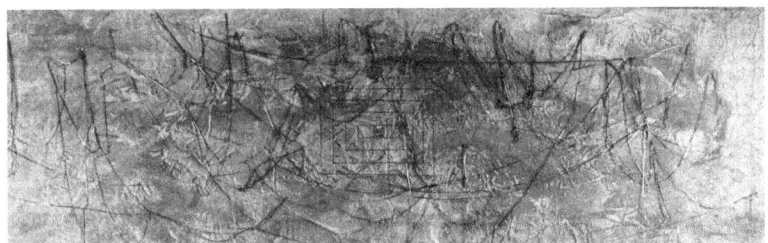

EXPOSED, 4ft. x 13ft., Mixed Media - 1996

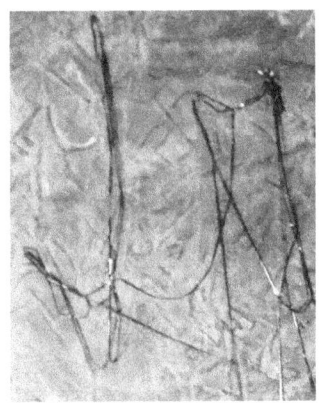 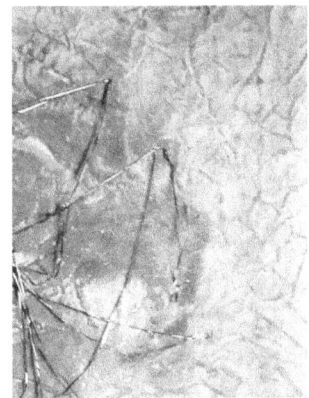

EXPOSED (close-ups) - 1996

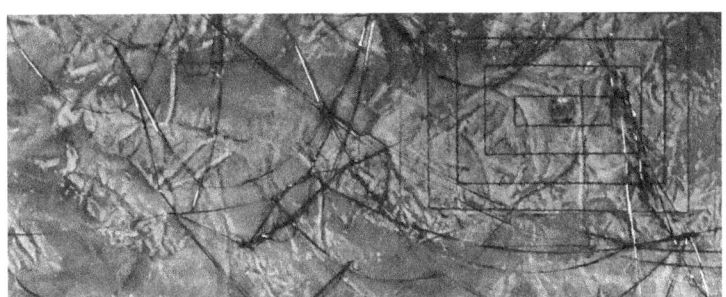

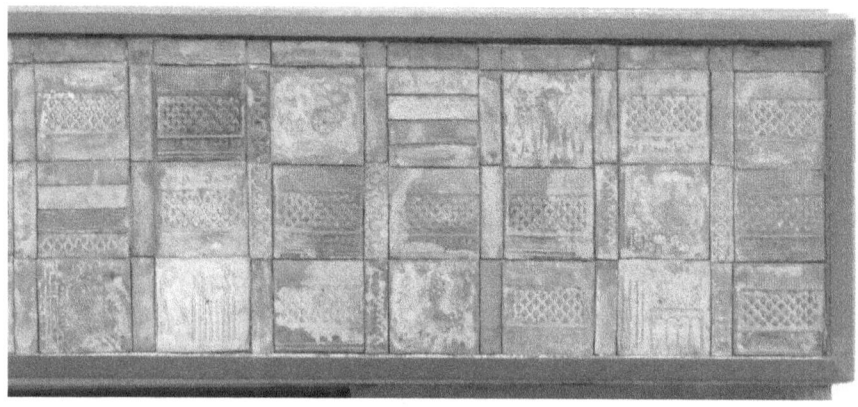

GRANADA - Ceramic Mural - 1992

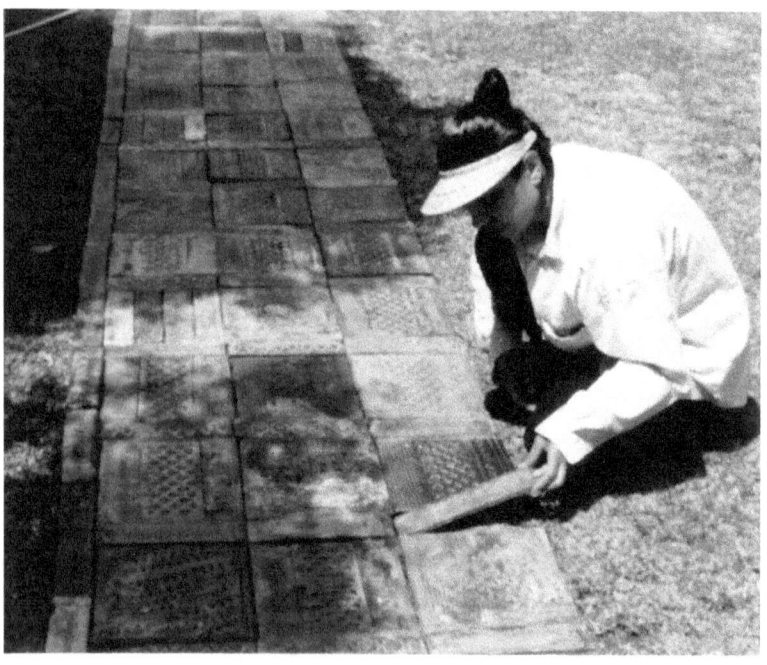

GRANADA - (Hanaa Al-Wardi Assembling the Granada Tiles) - 1992

"TEDDY BEARS FOR IRAQ" PROJECT - Photos during Iraq trip right after the first Gulf War

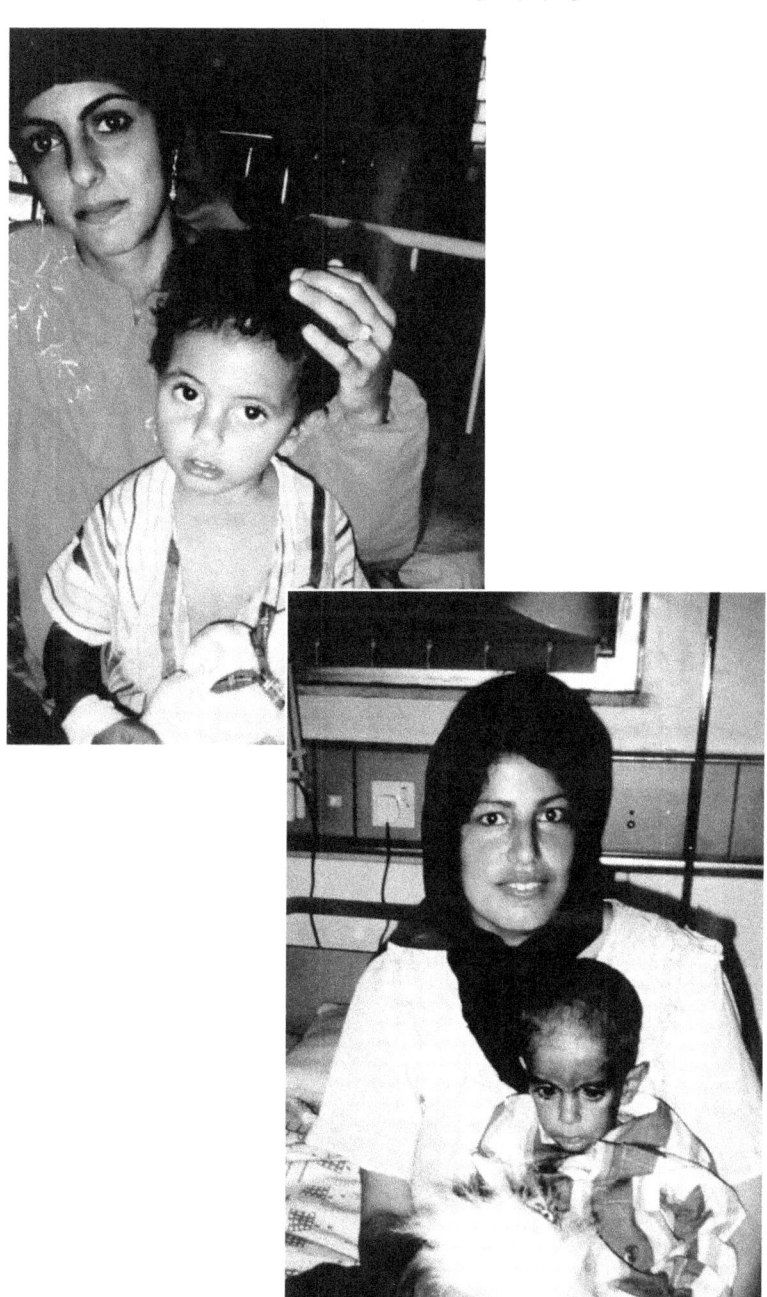

"TEDDY BEARS FOR IRAQ" PROJECT - Photos during Iraq trip right after the first Gulf War of 1992

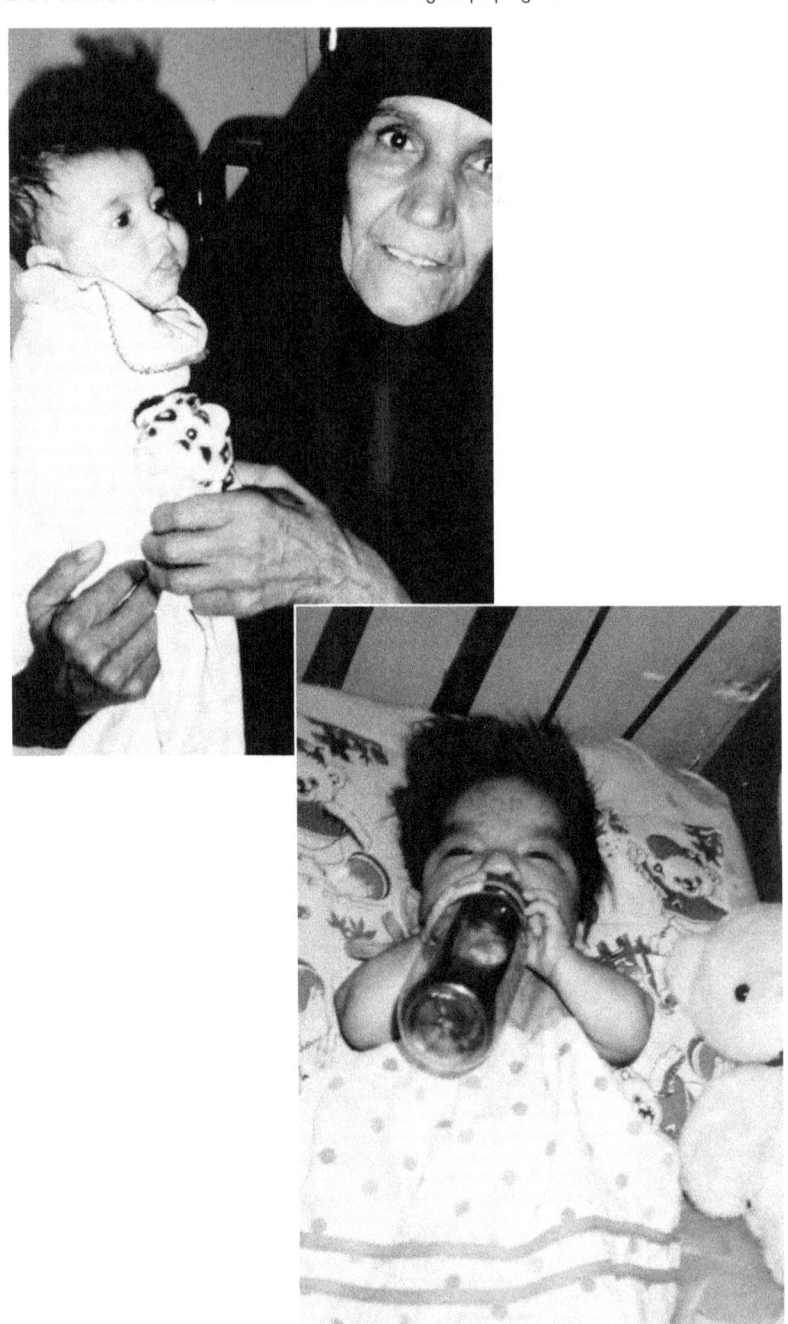

"TEDDY BEARS FOR IRAQ" PROJECT - Photos during Iraq trip right after the first Gulf War of 1992

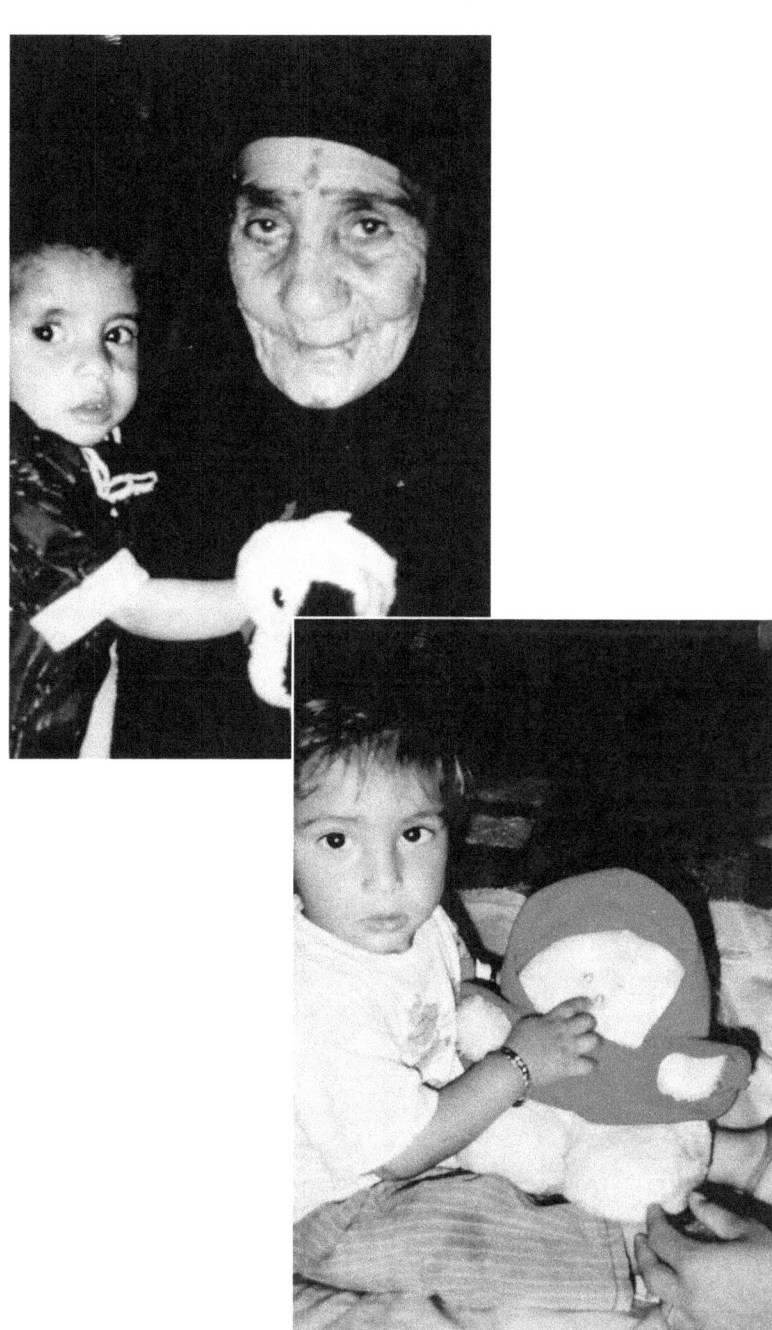

"TEDDY BEARS FOR IRAQ" PROJECT - Photos during Iraq trip right after the first Gulf War of 1992

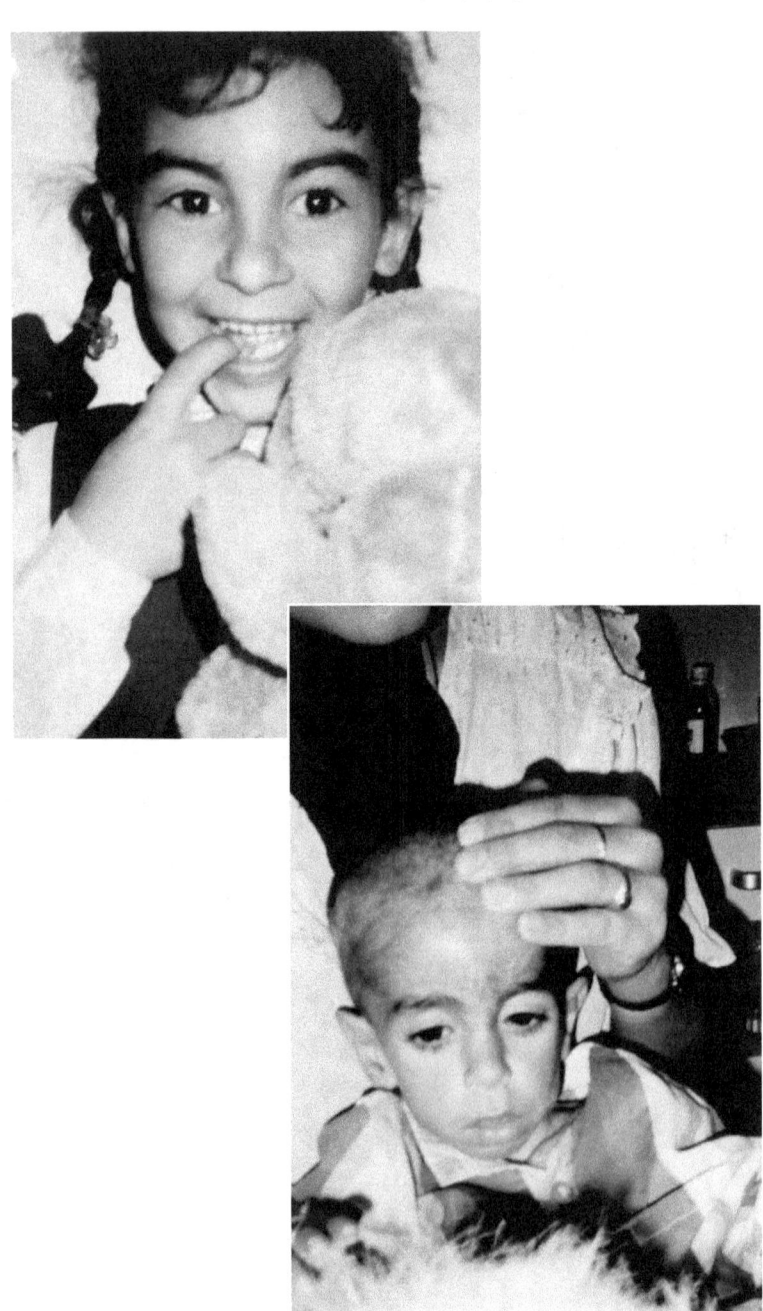

"TEDDY BEARS FOR IRAQ" PROJECT - Photos during Iraq trip right after the first Gulf War of 1992

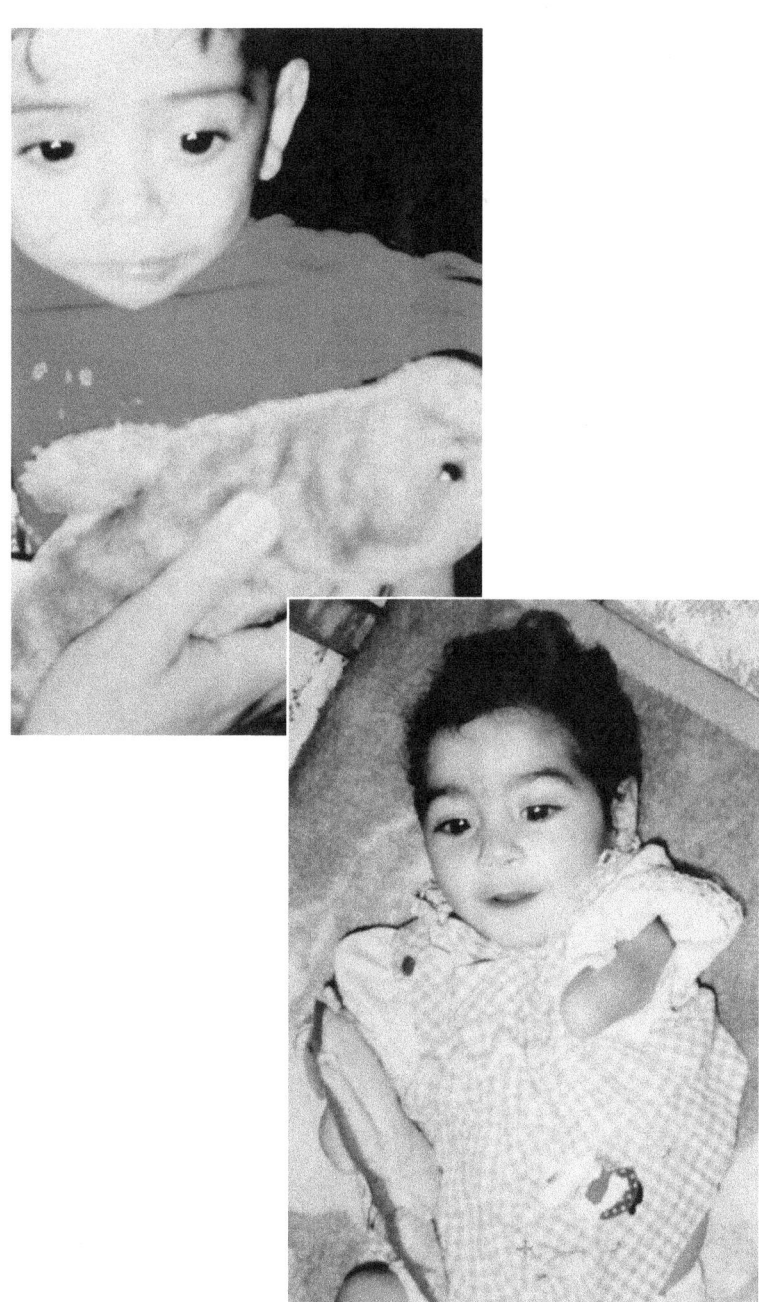

"TEDDY BEARS FOR IRAQ" PROJECT - Photos during Iraq trip right after the first Gulf War of 1992

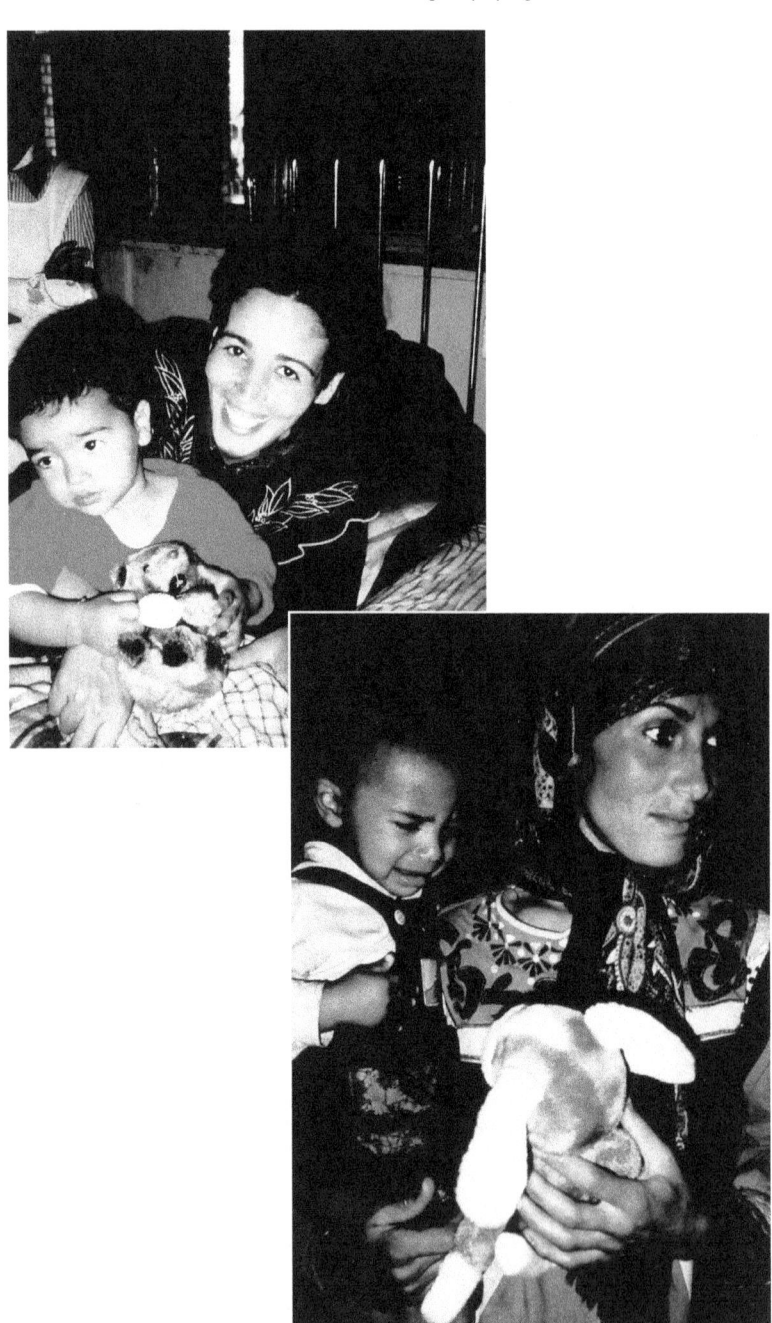

"TEDDY BEARS FOR IRAQ" PROJECT - Photos during Iraq trip right after the first Gulf War of 1992

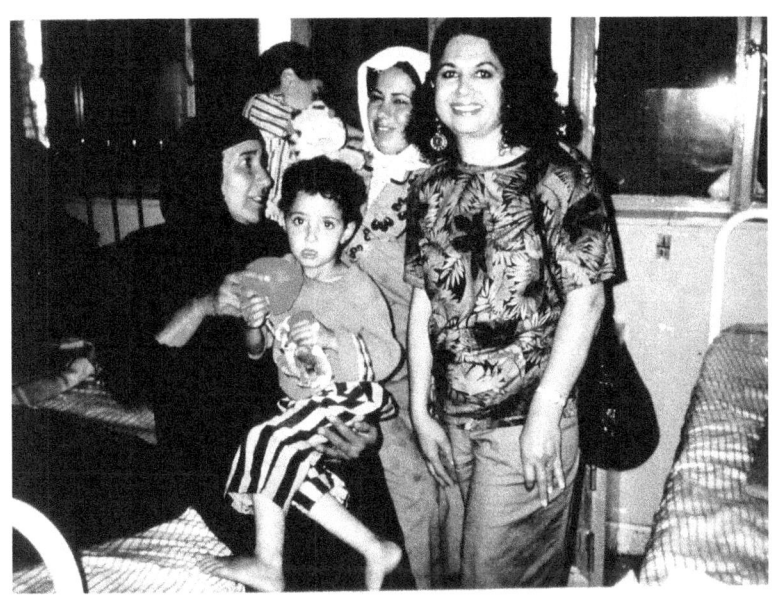

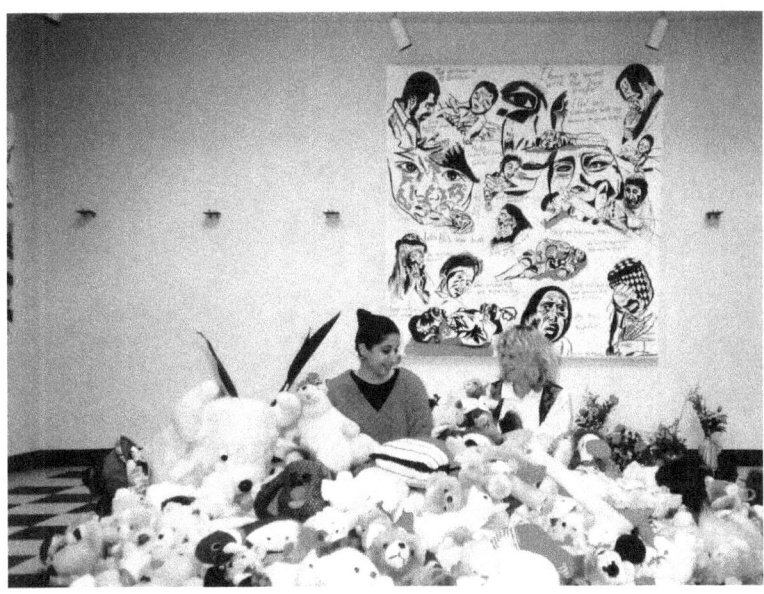

CLIPPINGS FROM VARIOUS ARTICLES

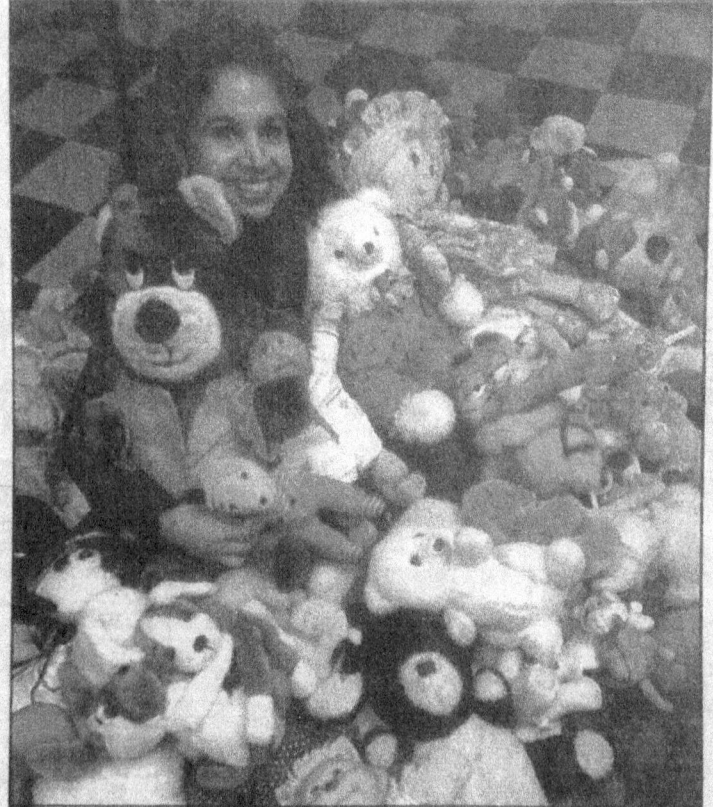

Traveling teddy bears

Staff Photo / Walt Mancini

Relief effort: Haana Al-Wardi is organizing to send medical goods and more than 2,000 stuffed animals to Iraqi children who are suffering from the effects of the Persian Gulf War. Al-Wardi owns an art gallery in Alhambra./**A-6**

CLIPPINGS FROM VARIOUS ARTICLES

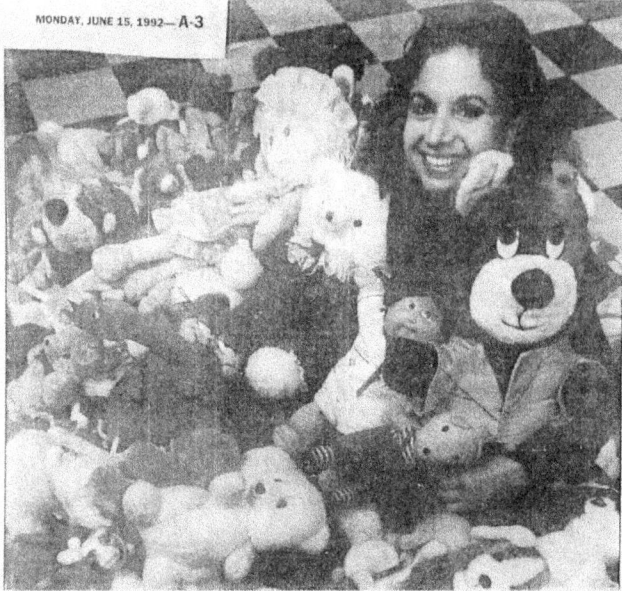

MONDAY, JUNE 15, 1992—A-3

File photo / Walt Mancini

Set free: Hanaa Al-Wardi, an Alhambra artist, poses with stuffed animals she took to Iraqi children in April, after getting government approval. The animals were detained for 59 days at Los Angeles International Airport because of sanctions imposed after Iraq invaded Kuwait.

Teddy bear blockade ends, artist delivers stuffed animals to Iraq

By Felicia Paik
Staff Writer

ALHAMBRA — After battling a United Nations-sponsored economic embargo and federal red tape for six months, Hanaa Al-Wardi finally got to do what she originally intended: deliver teddy bears to children in Iraq.

"It was a hard trip, but it was worth it," said Al-Wardi, an Alhambra artist who returned last month from a four-week tour of Baghdad. "When we saw the children's faces and their smiles, that was enough for us."

Beginning in October, Al-Wardi and Santa Barbara nurse Diane Judice collected more than 3,000 teddy bears and toys, 60 boxes of children's clothing and two tons of medical supplies as a Persian Gulf War relief effort.

The clothing and medicine were allowed for shipment — but not the teddy bears, which were detained for 59 days at Los Angeles International Airport because of sanctions imposed after Iraq invaded Kuwait.

At the end of March, a special order from the United States ended the teddy bear blockade, and Al-Wardi and Judice finally made their travel plans to Jordan and Baghdad.

"I'm a very spiritual person," said Judice, 36. "I never doubted that the bears would finally be able to go. I knew that with all the letters and phone calls I made to the U.S. Treasury and the United Nations we would finally get approval."

Al-Wardi and Judice left April 17 for Jordan. It took eight days for the shipment to clear customs in Amman. The two women then hired a driver and a 36-foot-long truck recommended by Catholic Relief Services to take them and their goods through the country to Iraq.

"It took us 26 hours to get there, and we slept in the truck because the driver told us it was unsafe to drive through the night due to bandits," Al-Wardi said.

The women visited more than 35 hospitals, orphanages, foster homes and free clinics in Baghdad and distributed the toys and other goods.

"It was very emotional for me," said Al-Wardi, who moved to the United States from Baghdad 22 years ago. "I couldn't believe we had finally made it. The mothers and children were so happy to receive the toys. Although they certainly don't have enough, they are used to receiving medicine."

The two women said although the Iraqis have inadequate medicine for heart ailments or stomach ulcers and no facilities to provide chemotherapy to children who have cancer, they weren't shocked by what they saw.

"Both of us had prepared for the worst," Al-Wardi said. "We were expecting to see dead people in the street and starving children. But it wasn't as bad as we expected."

Al-Wardi said she is working on a new exhibit for her gallery on West Main Street.

"I took about 400 slides while in Iraq, and I hope to incorporate them in an exhibit about the children of war or mothers and children," she said. "I'm glad I went because now the mourning is over."

Judice is already at work on her next project, Teddy Bears for Los Angeles, for children living in the areas devastated by the recent riots.

"Just like in the war between the United States and Iraq, there is no listening going on here," Judice said. "We need to listen to all sides because there is partial truth to what every side sees."

53

CLIPPINGS FROM VARIOUS ARTICLES

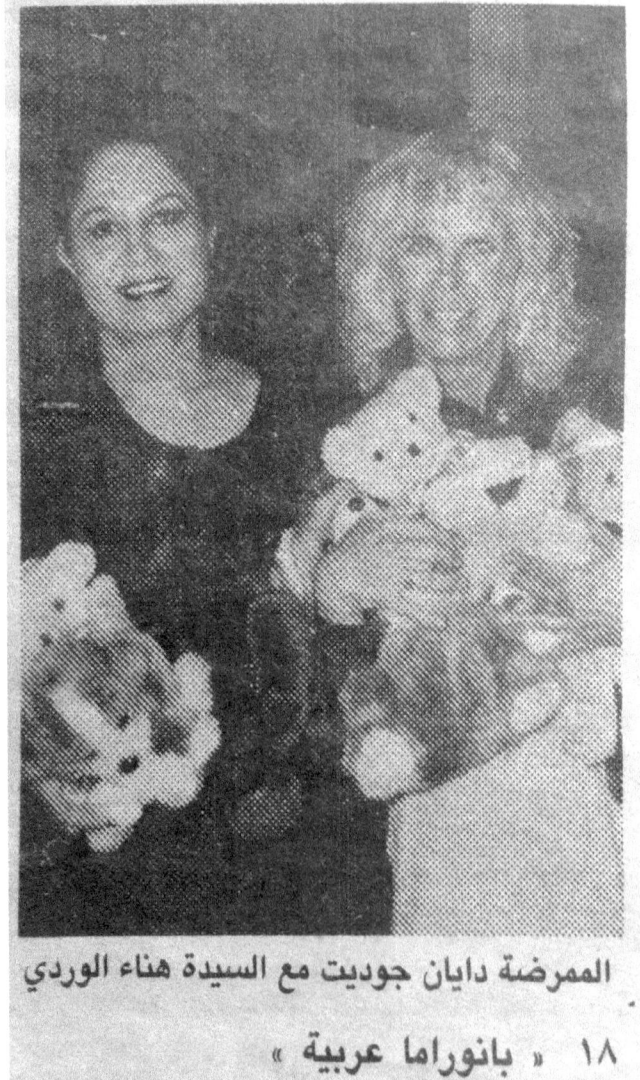

الممرضة دايان جوديت مع السيدة هناء الوردي

١٨ « بانوراما عربية »

CHAPTER 4

ART AND
PROBLEM
SOLVING

The creative art process by itself is full of problem solving and decision making. Eventually it will lead you to polish your skills and capabilities in problem solving, because you must think outside the box and not limit yourself with mainstream thinking, black and white solutions, or be stuck in one way of seeing things. By doing it over and over for a long time, it becomes a part of you. It's very important to have various solutions and approaches to finish the work you intend. This skill will lead you to real-life problem solving among families, friends and co-workers. Usually, artists are more flexible and willing to revise their thinking and plans. When they are faced with problems and obstacles, their brains think outside the mainstream. Also, artists usually self-reflect and experiment with different approaches to solve the problems they face.

you must think outside the box and not limit yourself with mainstream thinking, black and white solutions, or be stuck in one way of seeing things.

In my case, throughout my long career as an artist, when I make mistakes doing a specific project, I never feel disappointed or upset. I always work around it and revise it and make something totally different from my original intention. Usually the results are very pleasing. That makes me very happy and gives me a sense of great accomplishment. A change of direction is not bad; rather, it is an opportunity to explore other methods. All mistakes happen for a reason, so embrace them and do something with them. I am not stuck with one approach; I am open to other possibilities, and most of the time the result is a better outcome than the original thought. I contribute that approach to the art process. Indirectly condition your mind to be free and always think of other possibilities. If I feel that my subconscious mind is directing me to change course, I trust it totally.

A change of direction is not bad; rather, it is an opportunity to explore other methods.

On the other hand, sometimes when I make a mistake I leave it to remind myself not to do it again. Creating art, any kind of art-music, photography, dancing, poetry, etc. always allows you to express your inner feelings, thoughts and imaginations. It really is an extension or a bridge between your mind and your hand.

When you decide to do creative projects, you will encounter many challenges and decisions you have to resolve before you even start. You are challenged with all kinds of questions: What medium should I use? What color scheme should I use? What is the subject matter? You are so totally consumed by the decisions of the process, and that by itself will definitely shift your focus to the art and not on the stressful situation. Visual thinking and creative skills by themselves will help you to be more skillful in the process of problem solving by

Creating art, any kind of art-music, photography, dancing, poetry, etc. always allows you to express your inner feelings, thoughts and imaginations. It really is an extension or a bridge between your mind and your hand.

forcing you to constantly make choices about deciding how best to approach your art project. Your brain is thus in a very active mode and hypersensitive to ideas and fluid thinking, which usually leads you to solve the problem. Eventually it becomes second nature. You can finish the project or control the outcome and that by itself contributes a great deal to stress reduction and can elevate your confidence and self-esteem.

A Guggenheim study reveals the importance of art in problem solving. This "Learning Through Art" study was published in New York on June 2, 2010. For the first phase of the study, the Guggenheim's "Learning Through Art" (LTA) staff assembled an advisory team of artists, educators, and cognitive scientists to identify the problem-solving skills that visual arts can most powerfully teach, followed by two years of research conducted by an evaluation consultant team from Randy Korn and Associates. The final year focused on the analysis and dissemination of the findings.

The two years of the study's data collection efforts involved measures that were both quantitative and qualitative in nature. The study included the observation of artists teaching in eighteen classrooms, observations of twenty-five student case studies, questionnaires, interviews with eighteen participating classroom teachers, and one-on-one interviews in which 447 test and control students were given an art-based problem-solving task and were asked to describe their process in completing it. The results of this research revealed that students receiving LTA instruction scored higher in three out of the six skills of problem solving as defined by the study: flexibility space (the ability to revise or rethink one's plan when faced with challenges); connections of ends and aims (the ability to reflect on whether one's final work of art met the intended goals); and resources recognition (the ability to identify additional materials that could be applied to the completion of the project). The three other skill areas were identified as imagining, experimentation, and self-reflection.

"The study conducted by the Learning Through Art program demonstrates that arts education helps develop the skills necessary to persistently and adaptively work through problems," said Kim Kantani, deputy director and Gail Engelberg director of education for the, Solomon R. Guggenheim foundation. The study reports, "By asking the students to think like artists, we are impacting the 21st century skills in encouraging a Zen approach to problems with

The study reports, "By asking the students to think like artists, we are impacting the 21st century skills in encouraging a Zen approach to problems with creativity and analytic thoughts rather than just recitation of facts."

creativity and analytic thoughts rather than just recitation of facts."

The art of problem solving represents the Guggenheim's second major U.S. Department of Education-funded study of Learning through Art. In 2003, the Guggenheim received its first art in education model development and dissemination grant from the US Department of Education for completion of the ground breaking three-year research initiative that realized that LTA improved students' literacy and critical thinking. The full research reports and executive summaries of the art problem solving and teaching literacy through art studies are available at www.learningthroughart.org.

The ground breaking three-year research initiative that realized that LTA improved students' literacy and critical thinking.

CHAPTER 5

THINK LIKE AN
ARTIST

W hat I mean is, don't get stuck in problems and feel desperate. Don't think that there is no way out. Think like an artist! Artists are more flexible in their thinking and more accepting of controversial issues and they see many shades of colors. Usually, they think outside of the box and feel freer to explore other methods and ways to solve any difficulties and obstacles they face.

Artists also ask other people for their opinions, input, suggestions and critical analysis. This type of feedback is surprisingly inspiring and opens even more approaches, methods and solutions.

Also, you can program your subconscious mind to dream of ways and solutions to your problems. This has served me well; anything I ask my subconscious mind clearly and specifically three times before I go to sleep, I dream about. It might not be exactly the same, but it's symbolically right on.

Actually, my subconscious mind helped me a great deal and directed me on how to approach writing this book and gave me many hints and suggestions and ways to proceed. Any time I get stuck, my subconscious mind reminded me of experiences that helped me focus on writing, and I have included them in this book.

Think like an artist! Artists are more flexible in their thinking and more accepting of controversial issues and they see many shades of colors. Usually, they think outside of the box and feel freer to explore other methods and ways to solve any difficulties and obstacles they face.

I always go to my subconscious mind and it never fails me. It's really an amazing source of information. It is like my own encyclopedia and it is all mine and accessible to me whenever I need it.

On the conscious level, you are very rigid and normally affected by your surroundings, your environment, your family and friends and interference from people around you. However, when you go to your subconscious mind, it's all yours while you sleep; nobody bothers you. It's your own and you can program it and it is under your command. I call it my wonderful GPS and I can use it anytime I want to solve my problems. It's like I have my own private therapist at my command. Programming your subconscious is a very powerful tool. Use it.

I always go to my subconscious mind and it never fails me. It's really an amazing source of information. It is like my own encyclopedia and it is all mine and accessible to me whenever I need it.

As a Master of Fine Arts student in the nineties, I used to observe my colleague's work and try to find connections between their art, personality and background. One specific young artist caught my attention. This artist used to create installations by building large chicken coops and then placing chickens in it. The cage was filled with straw, water, feed and other things for the chickens to live on. When the chicken laid eggs, she used to withhold the food. To my horror and everybody else's, the chickens started eating their own eggs. I just saw it once and felt very stressed and upset.

I never spoke to the artist directly. I asked my classmates about the artist and I was told that this young artist had horrible, dark experiences in her life. She was trying to purge all of her hate, pain and nightmares and transferring them into her installation for the whole world to see. Maybe she hoped someone would come and help her. Or maybe she has already helped heal herself or at least eased her pain through her expressive art.

She was trying to purge all of her hate, pain and nightmares and transferring them into her installation for the whole world to see.

CHAPTER 6

WHEN THINGS FALL APART, LEAN ON ART

Personally speaking, when I encounter stressful situations, I always lean on artistic activities. Art is my best friend. It has served me very well throughout my life. I can express anything I want: express it with colors, subject matter, texture, content, and the materials I use. When I am sad, the colors I favor are usually dark colors, gloomy and cloudy. The subject matter usually tends to be depressing or angry and pessimistic, but this is normal; your body is trying to get rid of stress and pressure. Then you feel much better. It's a very necessary natural process to go through to purge the stress away, to paint your stress away. It is a process of cleansing your system and detoxifying your mind.

By using collections of specific photos or harsh objects (for example wood, glass, metal, pennies, coins, branches, twigs, rocks and crushed stones) and by assembling a collage project to express your feelings, you can tell a story about a political situation you don't like, or a very tough encounter from a traumatic experience in your life. Personally, when

> *To paint your stress away, "is a process of cleansing your system and detoxifying your mind."*

I'm happy, usually the colors I choose for my projects tend to be beautiful, bright and with a translucent and shimmery hue. It really reflects my mood. When I look at the finished work, it feels like it is singing to me and that is a very uplifting experience and a great accomplishment.

THE MEANING OF COLORS IN THE ART EXPRESSION PROCESS

Blue: calming, lowers heart rate, reduction of appetite, induces tranquility, represents dependability

Green: induces harmony, balance, security, stability, hope, growth, healing ability, visually pleasing

Purple: Regal, dignified, civilized, creative

Brown: warm, earth, basic, evokes a sense of time and nostalgia

Gray: Sense of peace, maturity

Red: Boosts energy, life, vitality, love, power, attracts attention, heightens appetite

Yellow: cheerful, happy, ready and motivated

White: safety, purity, innocence and simplicity

Black: dignity, grief

THE ABSTRACT ARTIST'S APPROACH

When I go to my studio to work on any project, usually I approach my art intuitively, spontaneously. I depend heavily on my intuition and I trust it totally, so whatever comes is fine with me. I don't title my work until it is finished. Then I stare at it and wait for it to tell me what I should call it. I have to take this approach to understand my inner feelings.

When I look at the finished work, it feels like it is singing to me and that is a very uplifting experience and a great accomplishment.

If you take this approach, you will be very happy with the results, because it is a very real and truthful approach.

My artwork usually tells stories. Each one tells a different story. The viewer doesn't know what the story is, and because it is abstract, I am the only one who knows. The viewer really doesn't know unless they ask me. I want them to use their imagination to interpret the meaning of the piece, but I do know the meaning. I don't follow any rules; I just go in and take the plunge. Mostly, I'm very happy with the results. I listen to my inner feelings and stop when they tell me I'm done.

In the mid-nineties, I created a piece and named it *Oil Spills and Greed*. I used a lot of copper pennies to symbolize greed. I love this piece, and I think it is very strong. But when one viewer saw it, he loved it and thought to buy it to bring him more money and prosperity. He was a business man and wanted to hang it in his office. I felt so disappointed and I told him about the meaning behind the piece. He changed his mind. I just couldn't sell it to someone who didn't get the meaning.

I don't follow any rules; I just go in and take the plunge. Mostly, I'm very happy with the results. I listen to my inner feelings and stop when they tell me I'm done.

I use different media; I don't like to be restricted to one medium to express what I feel. It all depends on my mood; sometimes I work solely in ceramics, sometimes in photography, sometimes painting, sometimes assembly and lately designing and making jewelry. Even the jewelry pieces are different from one to another, and each one tells a story because of the stones I use. The centerpieces are things from all over the world I collected decades ago, like beads from all over the world and some I assembled or fabricated myself. My jewelry pieces are mainly necklaces. Each piece is very different from the others in color, texture, design and content.

My necklaces are *"Wow Pieces."* Each piece has its own character and personality. When you wear one, you will be noticed immediately. To view my jewelry collection, please visit www.hagallery.com.

I call my art *"intuitive art"* because it is not based on premeditated or preconceived ideas. It usually starts as a seed and flourishes into a beautiful tree. On the other hand, for the political exhibits, usually I have general idea, but the subject is not clear in my mind at the beginning. The subject usually crystallizes and becomes more focused when I listen to the news or read the newspaper and political magazines to get some substance and inspiration for the exhibit, and then I interpret the subject my own way.

I call my art "intuitive art" because it is not based on premeditated or preconceived ideas. It usually starts as a seed and flourishes into a beautiful tree.

EXAMPLES OF JEWELRY MADE AND DESIGNED BY HANAA AL-WARDI

1983-2014

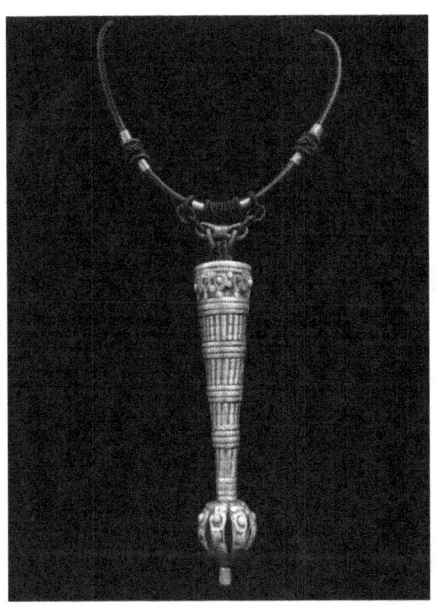

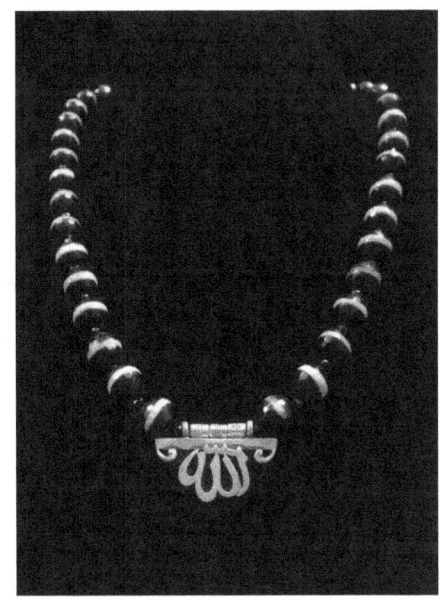

EXAMPLES OF JEWELRY MADE AND DESIGNED BY HANAA AL-WARDI

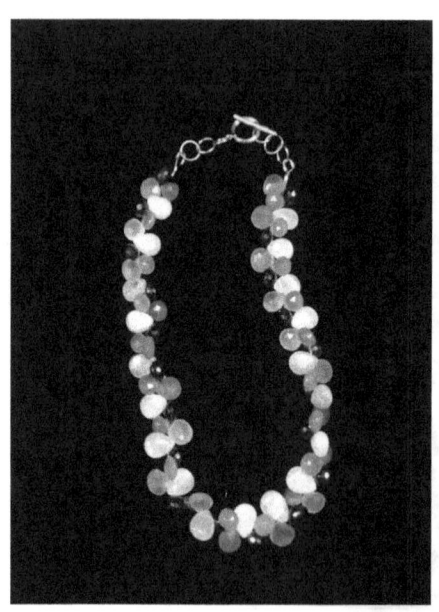

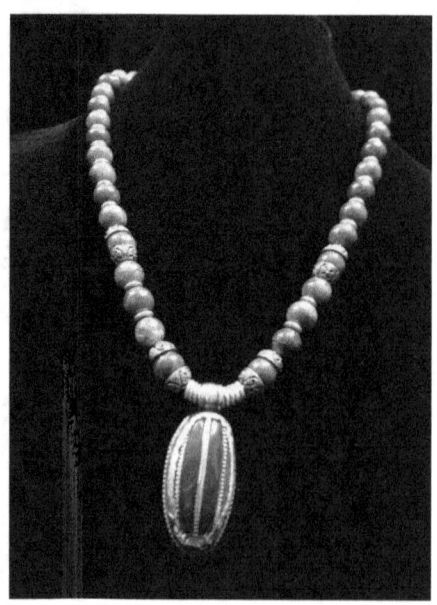

EXAMPLES OF JEWELRY MADE AND DESIGNED BY HANAA AL-WARDI

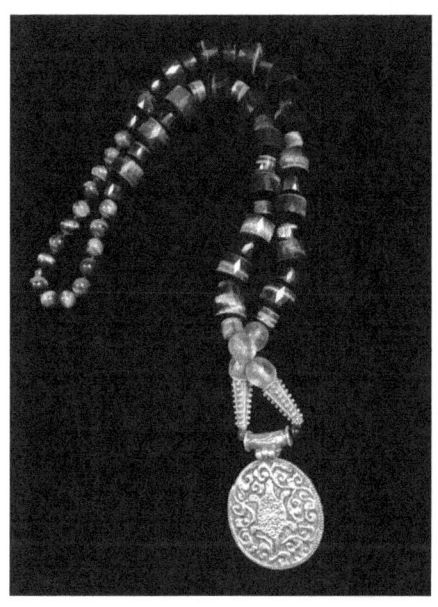

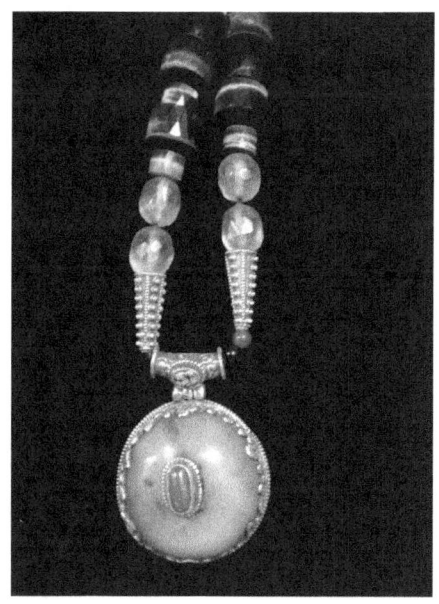

EXAMPLES OF JEWELRY MADE AND DESIGNED BY HANAA AL-WARDI

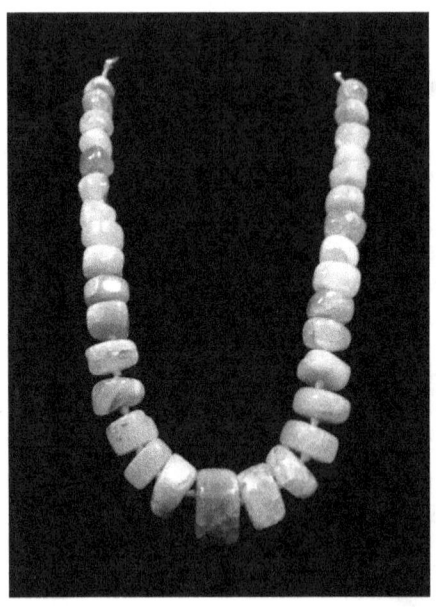

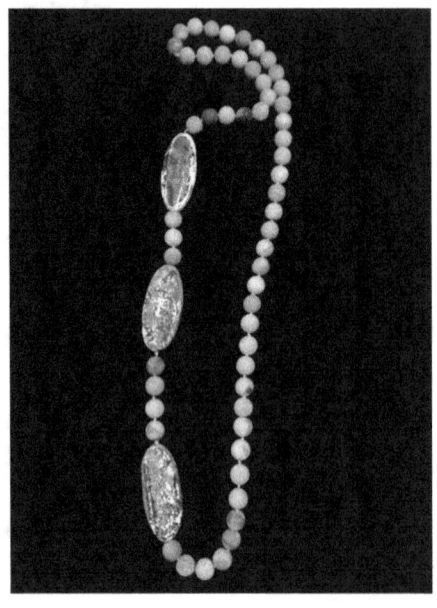

EXAMPLES OF JEWELRY MADE AND DESIGNED BY HANAA AL-WARDI

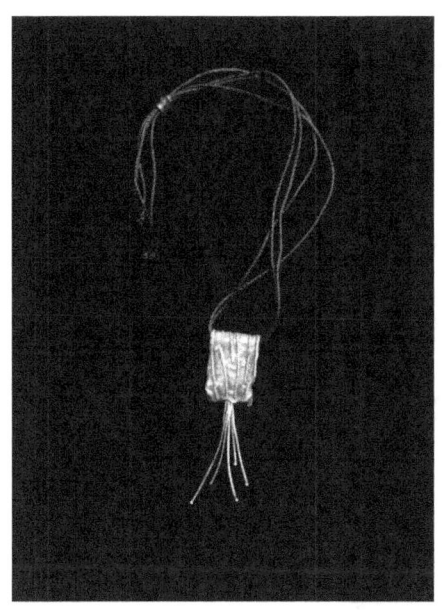

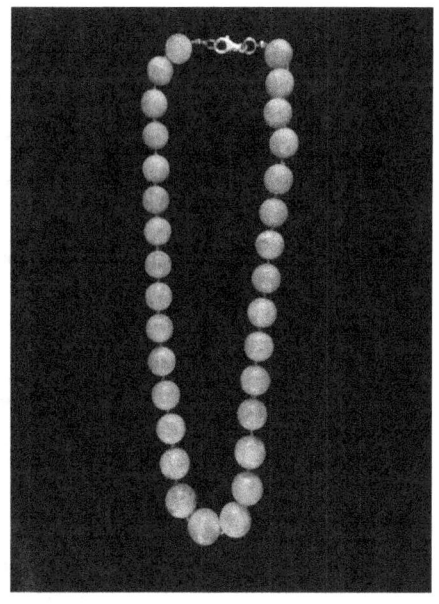

EXAMPLES OF JEWELRY MADE AND DESIGNED BY HANAA AL-WARDI

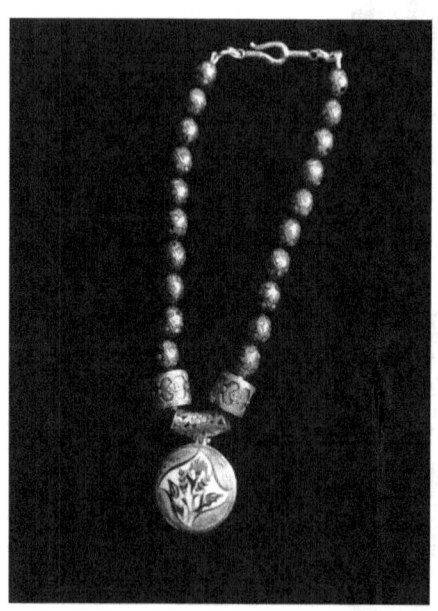

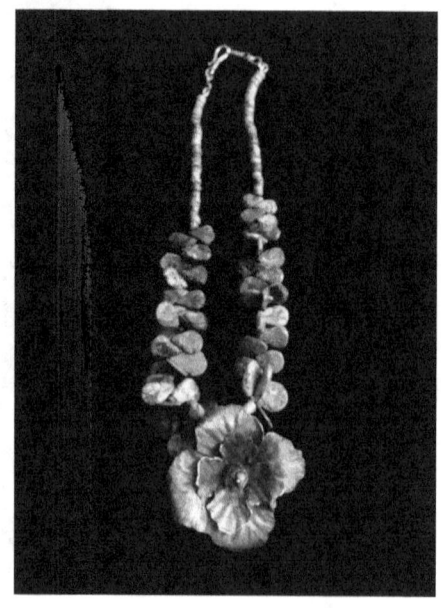

EXAMPLES OF JEWELRY MADE AND DESIGNED BY HANAA AL-WARDI

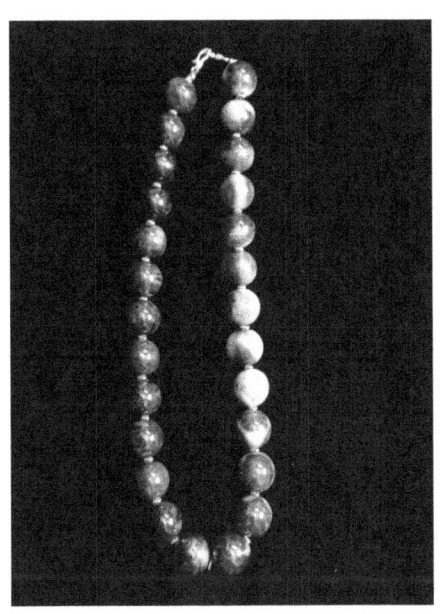

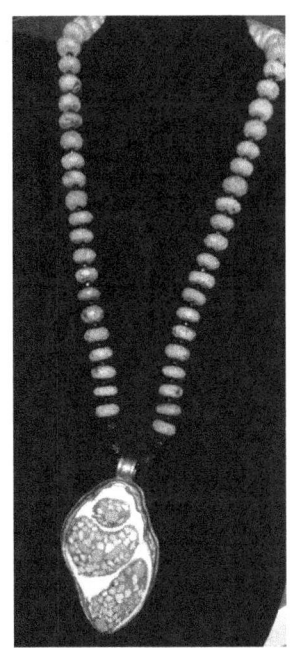

EXAMPLES OF JEWELRY MADE AND DESIGNED BY HANAA AL-WARDI

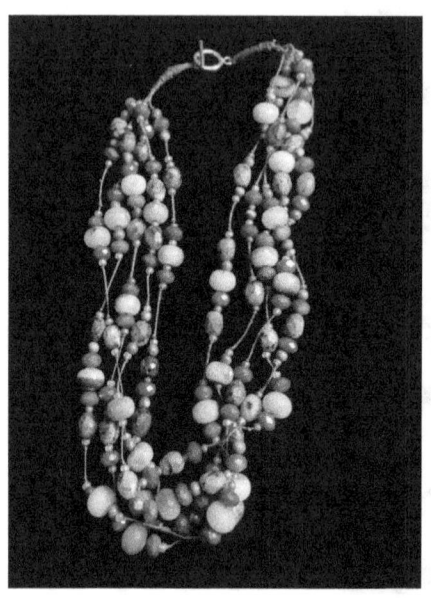

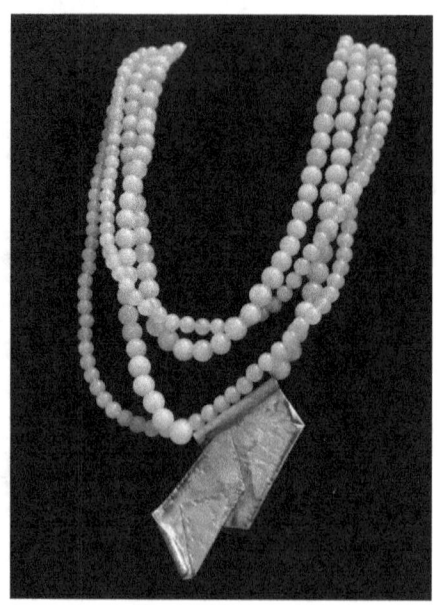

EXAMPLES OF JEWELRY MADE AND DESIGNED BY HANAA AL-WARDI

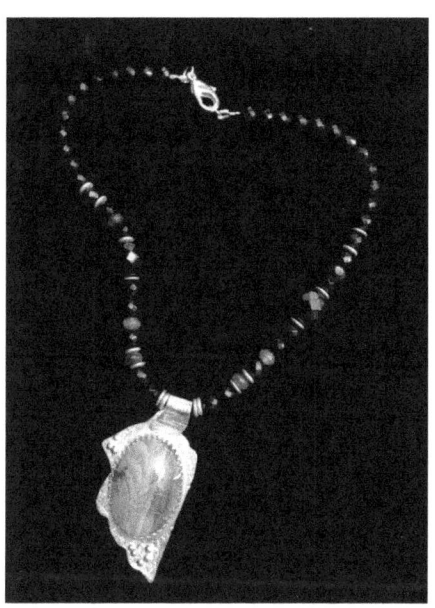

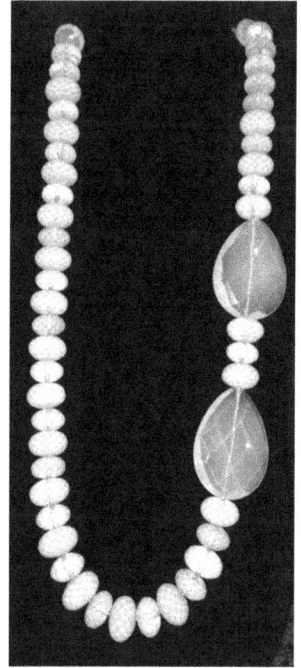

PAINT YOUR
STRESS AWAY

CHAPTER 7

THE
ART
CONNECTION

Medical science has finally started to incorporate art therapy into valid and tangible treatment programs for patients with all kinds of illnesses. More and more studies are showing that the benefit of art therapy is that the patients are encouraged to see and explore the images they create, distracting them from their health issues. It also helps them to become more self-aware, express their fears, anxieties and other emotions that may be difficult to verbalize.

More and more physicians are realizing that art therapy, like physical therapy, has tremendous value to the recovery of their patients. Many are referring their adult patients with cancer to art therapy to manage their pain and symptoms and to facilitate the psychological changes associated with the loss, change, and uncertainty of cancer and other diseases.

Stress is especially dangerous for those with cancer. It has even been tied to a lower survival rate. A new study suggests that mindfulness art can help decrease anxiety among this group. Creative arts therapy, in addition to a mindfulness training program, seems to provoke actual brain changes linked with decreased stress in women with breast cancer. The study was published in the *Stress and Health* Journal.

Creative arts therapy, in addition to a mindfulness training program, seems to provoke actual brain changes linked with decreased stress in women with breast cancer. The study was published in the Stress and Health Journal.

"This type of expressive and meditation program has never before been studied for physiological impact and the correlation of that impact to improvement in stress and anxiety," study researcher Dr. Daniel Monti, M.D., the director of the Jefferson Myrna Brind Center of Integrative Medicine, said in a statement.

The study included eighteen people with breast cancer who received their diagnosis sometime between three years before the study and six months before the study. None of the participants were in active treatment for their cancer. At the start of the study, they were asked to fill out a checklist of ninety symptoms, and they also underwent FMRI (Functional Magnetic Resonance Imaging) as they did a neutral task, a stressor task, and a meditative task.

Some were assigned to take a mindfulness-based therapy course, while others were assigned to just take an education course, both for eight weeks. The mindfulness-based therapy course included lessons on mindful yoga, mindful breathing, emotional awareness, etc., as well as art activities where they were able to express themselves emotionally.

After the eight-week period, the study participants filled out the symptom checklist again, and also underwent the brain scan again.

Researchers found that the study participants who were assigned to the mindfulness-based therapy course showed changes in the brain, mainly in the areas controlling stress, the reward and emotion. Specifically, they experienced more cerebral blood flow in the left insula, amygdala and hippocampus region of the brain.

The study published in the *Stress and Health Journal* concluded that the participants in the mindfulness-based art therapy course also experienced less anxiety and stress, according to their responses to the symptom checklist.

Researchers found that the study participants who were assigned to the mindfulness-based therapy course showed changes in the brain, mainly in the areas controlling stress, the reward and emotion.

At Memorial Sloan-Kettering Cancer Center, they have an excellent counseling and art therapy program for cancer patients. The patients at the Evelyn H. Lowder Breast Center participate in an art therapy program that includes drawing, painting, and other media. In this program, patients can work with trained art therapists in a safe, private, and relaxing environment to find ways to express their experiences through art. No prior art experience is required. Regardless of their stage of treatment or recovery, the patients are welcomed at the art therapy open studio with their family members, friends and caregivers.

The benefit of art therapy is that the patients are encouraged to see and explore the images they create through art therapy that can distract them from their health issues. It also helps them to become more self-aware, express their fears, anxieties and other emotions that may be difficult to verbalize. Also, it helps in communication and interaction between patients and caregivers. It lessens their stress, builds self-esteem, improves their quality of life, and gives them comfort, freedom and hope.

At the art therapy program, patients can use a variety of materials to express their feelings: watercolors, paint, pencils, crayons and pastels, collage materials, color paper, origami or tissues, acrylic paints, drawing instruments like charcoal, graphite pencils, pens and ink. They also use molding clay and scratch board. Also, the staff at the hospital encourages patients to think and reflect on their hopes and dreams and showcase their work to the public.

PAINT YOUR
STRESS AWAY

CHAPTER 8

ART THERAPY

Art therapy goes way back. Before there were anti-depressants, there were cave drawings. Using art to express yourself has its roots in the theories of Freud and Jung, who both believed in the power of imagery to tap into the thoughts, memories and feelings of a person.

The use of symbolism in dreams can help to uncover unconscious thoughts and feelings and to access the inner feelings and communication much faster through the arts than the spoken word.

In the early 1900s, Margaret Naumburg, an educator, with her total dedication and commitment to the power of art therapy for the healing of so many conditions, helped move art therapy into a recognized profession to aid the emotional development of children. She brought art therapy into the public eye, and in 1969, the American Association of Art Therapy was formed.

Art therapy has been a valuable part of mental health services since 1945, when it was mainly and originally implemented by Veteran Administration hospital to help the returning Veterans of World War II.

By the eighties, the application of art therapy became widely used to treat many stressful situations that many people face on a daily basis, at home and at work.

The following list includes some of them:

1. Insufficient sleep
2. Lack of exercise
3. Mothers overwhelmed by responsibilities
4. Commuting
5. Work place incivility
6. Chronic pain
7. Lack of job security
8. Shift work hours

9.   Long work hours

10. Toxic bosses

11. Deadlines

12. High expectations

13. Unhappy relationships

14. Overwhelming responsibilities

15. Pressure to perform

16. Traumatic experience

17. Abusive treatment at home

18. Unsupportive partners

19. Emotional deprivation

20. Care givers

21. Death in the family

22. Indoor air quality

When you are bombarded with at least two of the above stressful situations, art therapy can be a very helpful tool to address your mental and physical wellbeing.

PROVEN HEALTH BENEFITS

Art therapy helps healing in various ways. First, the aesthetic quality of the work produced can lift a person's mood, boost self-awareness and improve self-esteem. Second, research shows that physiological functions such as heart rate, blood pressure and breathing become more rhythmic, deep and slow when people are deeply involved in an activity they enjoy. The focused attention required is much like a meditative state. In addition, making art also provides the ability to shift your moods very quickly and release anger and unhappiness almost instantaneously. Also, it gives you the opportunity to exercise your eyes and hands, improve hand-eye coordination, and stimulate new neurological pathways between the brain and the hands.

Because art therapy uses a language other than words, it is often employed in treating patients with physical or emotional illnesses who have difficulty talking about their fears and hopes, or about their anger and other strong emotions. The creation of art helps people get in touch with thoughts and feelings that are often hidden from the conscious mind.

Making art also provides the ability to shift your moods very quickly and release anger and unhappiness almost instantaneously.

Usually, an art therapist works in a hospital setting or private art sessions that take place on a one-on-one basis or in a small group or in a medical clinic. Usually, the art therapist provides a suitable place to work, gives some technical advice and guidance on materials, and provides serene, relaxing background music, a well-ventilated space and a critique on the patient's progress.

Knowing the background of the patient is usually very important to help understand their conditions or probable situations or illnesses so the art therapist can tailor a program for that individual. Also, the timing should be flexible and accommodating to the patient's needs. There should not be back-to-back sessions. There should be no pressure, and it should be a very pleasurable experience that they look forward to in order to unwind, feel good and feel hopeful. Usually, art therapy should last for six months or longer to be helpful. Since powerful thoughts and feelings can surface through art therapy, it is essential that the therapist be a qualified practitioner.

The art therapist should be a trained artist with additional art therapy credentials. The American Art Therapy Association recommends that an art therapist should meet the following requirements:

- A Bachelor's Degree with at least 15 semester credits in Studio Art and 12 semester credits in Psychology.
- A Master's Degree in Art Therapy.
- One year of post-graduate work under the

supervision of a registered art therapist.

The primary health benefits are stress reduction, reduced pain, reduction of the symptoms of various diseases and other stress-related ailments.

Usually, art therapy sessions last for seventy-five minutes each. There are different types of art therapy to choose from. The fees are usually paid by the patients. Most health insurance policies do not cover art therapy.

Art therapy sessions can be practiced in many other settings other than hospitals, such as:

- Art studios
- Support groups
- Psychiatric centers
- Schools
- Drug and alcohol rehabilitation programs
- Nursing homes
- Medical and forensic institutions
- Community outreach programs
- Wellness centers
- Corporate structures

Art therapy can also be used as a treatment for behavioral problems. It is frequently part of inpatient psychological treatment programs, including those for drug and alcohol abuse.

Patients recovering from trauma or serious injury often find art therapy particularly beneficial, as do people with a chronic illnesses, such as Parkinson's or Alzheimer's disease. In addition to these uses, art therapy can also help people with a serious or terminal illness to create a tangible record of their thoughts and emotions.

PAINT YOUR
STRESS AWAY

THE PRACTICAL APPLICATION OF ART THERAPY FOR DIFFERENT PHYSICAL AND MENTAL CONDITIONS

ATTENTION DEFICIT HYPERACTIVITY DISORDER (ADHD)

Art therapy is becoming widely used and accepted as an alternative form of treatment for depression, anxiety and ADHD. It can be a truly wonderful approach to create intense improvement of stress, tension, depression and the anxiety that often accompanies ADHD.

Art therapy provides a way to gain insight and understanding through self-expression. The fears and other emotions that often accompany panic disorders can be hard to express through words alone, and the creative process of art therapy can help a person tap into and express deep feelings. Art therapy can be used with people who have anxiety and panic disorders to assist in reducing stress, improving self-esteem, building problem-solving skills, resolving turmoil and conflicts, relaxing and calming nerves, expressing feelings and experiences, developing ways to cope, working toward wellbeing, and staying motivated during the recovery process.

Engaging in creative endeavors on your own may be a great way to combat stress and practice self-care. But to get started in art therapy, you will need guidance from a qualified art therapist to help you in the healing process. Qualified art therapists are usually available in a variety of settings, including community agencies, private practices, hospitals, and clinics.

Engaging in creative endeavors on your own may be a great way to combat stress and practice self-care.

It is important when seeking out an art therapist that he or she has additional experience working with people with panic disorders. Usually, your doctor or therapist may be able to refer you to a licensed art therapist in your area.

Art therapy is a great tool for those with ADHD, as it allows a person to express feelings, emotions, and release energy through their hands. Any time ADDers can do something free-flowing and unstructured is wonderful, and art is a really fantastic way to do this. I have read a lot about art therapy, but few have touched on the importance of creating something positive with that energy.

People with ADHD usually benefit a great deal from positive art activities like drawing, sketching, cartoons and coloring, because it induces very good changes in their mood state and happiness. The energy of painting and drawing releases positive energy through touching and movement, and that tremendous energy transforms into a positive mood state. On the other hand, people with negative feelings and depression can channel their raw emotion through creative art or by writing and drawing about their hopes, worries and sadness.

The energy of painting and drawing releases positive energy through touching and movement, and that tremendous energy transforms into a positive mood state.

Art therapy in ADHD cases is an alternative route for non-permanent stimulant medication and pricey behavioral therapy sessions. Art therapy can be implemented as a conjunctive treatment with medication. Art therapy guides children toward increased communication and expression and helps to decrease the severity and frequency of negative communication and defiant behaviors. One clinical study focused on both cognitive-behavioral therapy and art as therapy with a control group over the course of ten weeks. (See Resources List at the end of the book). The outcome of the study revealed that both cognitive behavioral therapy and art therapy had a positive effect on the behavior of children suffering from ADHD and other behavioral disorders and led to increased perception of control. The minimal, yet valuable art therapy research on ADHD and psychotropic medication suggests that standardized art therapy tools could be used to support ADHD treatment and research. The use of art in assessment seems to be particularly useful for children who might struggle with verbal assessments. With this information alone, why not give art therapy a chance to show what it can really do?

Art therapy can be beneficial to people of all ages, but it is especially useful for children and adolescents. Art is a natural form of communication for children because it is easier for them to express themselves visually rather than verbally. Art

Art therapy can be beneficial to people of all ages, but it is especially useful for children and adolescents.

making has also been shown to enhance cognitive abilities, improve social skills, and encourage self-esteem in school-age children.

Some experts believe that engaging in creative activities such as drawing, painting, listening to music and dancing helps children with ADHD calm down and focus better. Several studies suggest that music can help children with ADHD concentrate more easily, but more research needs to be done to confirm this. Still, some therapists and parents of children with ADHD say that these kids often do have an affinity for music and other kinds of artistic expression. Further, finding a creative outlet that allows a child to excel and express himself can be of great self-esteem booster.

For children with ADHD, artistic activity is greatly beneficial because it is fun, playful, and expressive, especially finger painting. Children love finger painting. They also love using leaves covered with paint and pressing them down on a piece of paper. Sun painting is also very interesting, and the kids love watching the colors change. If you use energetic music, while they paint, it will double the fun, and it is really a very uplifting activity. The kids will feel empowered and energized.

ALZHEIMER'S

It is widely acknowledged by health professionals that art therapy is very useful tool in helping people with Alzheimer's disease. It helps in triggering their forgotten memories and emotions, because art therapy focuses on other possibilities of untapped areas of the brain and helps to improve concentration. Art therapy emphasizes on the ability that is still available and can be developed rather than focusing on those that have been lost.

Alzheimer's attacks certain parts of the brain but leaves others intact and functioning, including some forms of memory and learning skills. Visual art provides an avenue to trigger these dormant memories and emotions and becomes a therapeutic experience for patients who are often unable to express themselves. Creative art can reunite even late-stage Alzheimer's sufferers with parts of their former selves.

Art therapy emphasizes the ability that is still available and can be developed rather than focusing on those that have been lost.

Artists for Alzheimer's.org and hilgos.org made a documentary called "I Remember Better When I Paint: Treating

Alzheimer's through Creative Arts," produced by French Connection Films and Hilgos Foundation. It can be seen on YouTube. The video is very touching and sensitive.

In one study conducted in a local U.S. hospital, thirty-nine patients with mild Alzheimer's disease were randomly assigned to either art therapy or learning therapy involving simple arithmetic once a week for twelve weeks. At the end of the study, the group who received art therapy showed significant improvements in vitality and quality of life, compared to the learning therapy group. The art activities used were very simple, mainly color by numbers, molding clay and photo collage.

Expression through art can become especially important as a person's ability to communicate through words deteriorates. When you try to engage your loved one in an art activity, first encourage them to look at pictures that are familiar to both of you and start a conversation about it. Also, choose an art project that is free form and easy to do. And don't be critical and strict about the colors. Remember, the picture is done when they say it is done. Familiar music that sparks memories is very helpful too.

The art activities used were very simple, mainly color by numbers, molding clay and photo collage.

BIPOLAR DISORDER

Bipolar disorder is also referred to as manic-depressive disorder due to the intense mood swings sufferers experience. Patients with bipolar disorder can become intentionally suicidal if the mood swings are severe enough. There are several means of therapy for bipolar disorder. One of them, art therapy, is gaining popularity as a treatment method during these phases. It is a common belief that the artwork of a person gives insights into her or his subconscious thought process. By extension, he or she can look into issues he or she may not consciously be aware of. If any repressed issues are brought to the surface, it is easier to confront them through the use of cognitive-behavioral therapy or a similar method. Art therapy is not a substitute for medication to control mental illness, but it may help someone who is struggling with a mental illness by boosting self-esteem and giving a sense of control. Art therapy is only one approach and should only be used as a supplement unless it proves more effective.

According to Mara McWilliams, an artist with bipolar disorder, her disorder benefited her and allowed her to tap into her creativity. Sometimes in a mania she can produce six inspired paintings in one week. Although bipolar disorder has many downfalls, you cannot ignore the benefits. She suggests that we too look at our lives and see where our disorder adds something special to our lives.

According to McWilliams, art therapy has been the one form of therapy that really opens her eyes to who she is and what she feels. Since finding this form of expression, she has healed in ways that she never thought would be possible for her. She used to be a cutter. One day, she decided that instead of slashing at herself with a razor, she would slash at the canvas in blood-colored paint with a brush. The release she felt was incredible. She was still able to express her rage and anger with all the intensity she needed by slicing away at the canvas instead of her body. Since she found that tool, she has not harmed herself. McWilliams said it sounds simple, and it really is.

ART BY BIPOLAR DISORDER PATIENTS

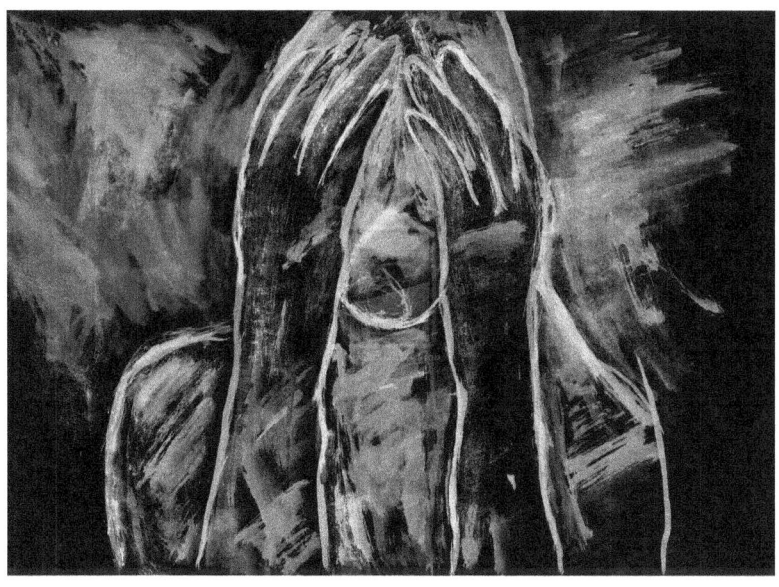

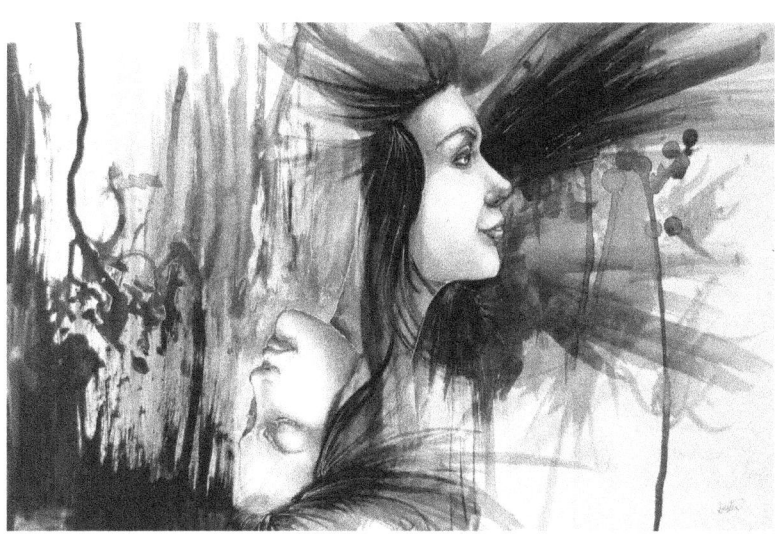

ART BY BIPOLAR DISORDER PATIENTS

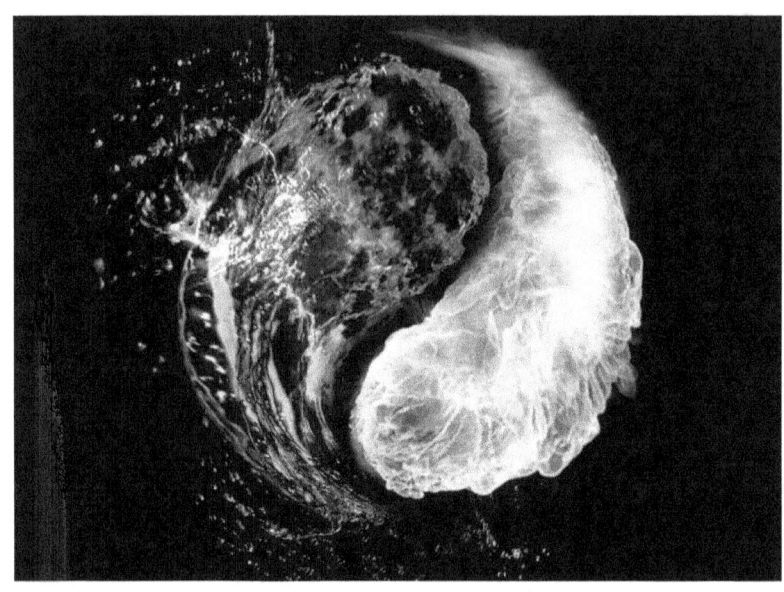

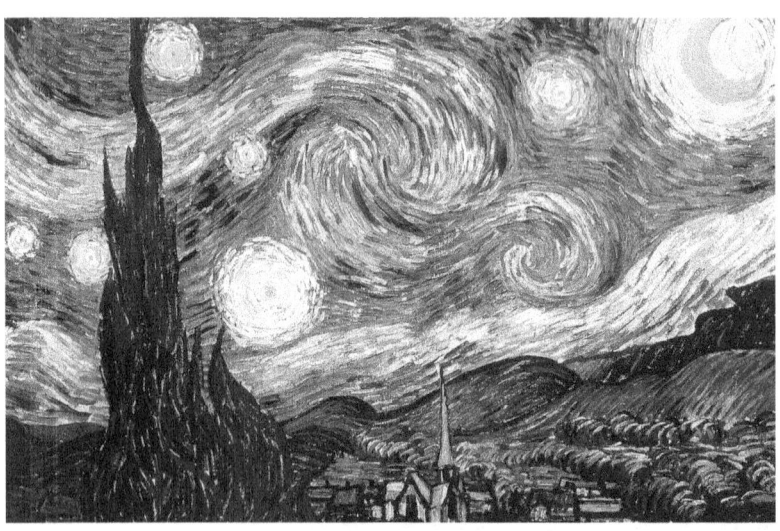

HEART HEALTH

Art therapy for heart health is particularly important in the reduction of inflammation, lowering blood pressure and lowering stress. Practicing art with meditation music, will double the benefit of heart healing. Art therapy now is recommended as part of the healing process to a healthy life after heart attack, to heal the scars and the damage to the heart muscle. Art therapy is also beneficial to those with chronic chest pain.

Even before you have a heart attack because of a blocked artery or arteries, usually you feel some discomfort in your chest, shallow breathing, weakness and severe exhaustion. These symptoms are your body telling you that there is something wrong and that you must pay attention.

Art therapy now is recommended as part of the healing process to a healthy life after heart attack.

Most heart illnesses are caused by stress or lack of sleep, which leads to physiological stress. Luckily, you can easily control and even reverse heart disease by managing your stress through art therapy. You can paint away your worries, disappointments in personal relationships, anger and failures in attaining your goals. When using a canvas or plain paper, you are emptying your stress, especially if you are journaling during the process.

Usually, when patients with heart disease get involved in the art process, they report that the chest pain and tightness lessen a great deal and feel much better than from using just medicine alone. Art is an effective temporary distraction from pain. Because of the widely acknowledged benefit of art therapy in easing pain and speeding recovery, many cardiologists recommend it along with medication.

When using a canvas or plain paper, you are emptying your stress, especially if you are journaling during the process.

From my personal experience, writing my inner thoughts on my art subjects is very freeing; usually I feel cleansed and at peace afterwards, which leads to de-stressing my mind, body and soul. Also, if I have any kind of pain, painting and getting involved in the process with music, will usually distract me from my pain.

An old patient at the clinic suffers from chronic pain all over his body. His pain includes chest pain, back pain, joint pain and migraines. When I asked him to describe how he deals with his pain, he replies: "I just ignore it and keep myself busy by trimming my rose bushes or looking through magazines, and by the way, I hate medicine." He advised me to never surrender to pain and find a way to conquer it instead.

Because of the widely acknowledged benefit of art therapy in easing pain and speeding recovery, many cardiologists recommend it along with medication.

Another patient used to come to the clinic for her severe migraines. She said that her employer is very demanding, disrespectful and unreasonable; he used to even ask her to answer the phone when she goes to the bathroom. She was under so much stress that it caused her to have chest pain and migraines on regular basis. She started taking medication for her migraines, her heart and her stress. After many months with little improvement, she asked me for suggestions and alternatives methods. I replied without any hesitation: "Quit your job and take art classes" at any adult school or community college and she did. After sometime, we were in touch again, and the patient shared with me that the art classes really helped. Her migraines subsided and her chest pain was gone!

POST-TRAUMATIC STRESS DISORDER

Art therapy can be beneficial to people of all ages, including adults who have emotional, cognitive, and/or physical disabilities. Our nation's veterans often return home with acute psychological or medical conditions that impair functioning, disrupt family relationships, and prevent their reentry into the workforce. Others may develop chronic disorders such as post-traumatic stress disorder (PTSD) that require months or even years of counseling or rehabilitation. For veterans who are receiving psychiatric care for PTSD and other emotional conditions, art therapy can be an effective form of treatment, even as an adjunct to other therapies or as a form of individual or group psychotherapy.

According to the report of the American Art Therapy Association on the subject of "Art Therapy, Post-Traumatic Stress Disorder, and Veterans," art therapy uses a wide variety of art-based techniques in the assessment and treatment of adults. For combat veterans of recent or previous conflicts, art therapy provides ways to express feelings and painful experiences that are difficult to express verbally.

As a form of psychotherapy, art therapy helps veterans communicate and resolve traumatic memories, relieve stress, and reduce symptoms of trauma-related conditions.

Art therapists encourage veterans to reflect on the meaning of their artwork to assist their psychological recovery, promote insight, and improve functioning.

For veterans in extended care facilities or hospitals, art therapy enhances quality of life by providing a meaningful creative vocation to increase self-esteem and sense of personal self-worth.

Based on their knowledge of art materials, human development, and physical, mental and emotional conditions, art therapists select specific drawing, painting, or sculpting activities to augment cognitive, psychological, and physical rehabilitation.

DID YOU KNOW?

Art therapy has been a valuable part of mental health services offered by the Veteran's Administration (VA) since 1945 when the Winter VA Hospital in Topeka, Kansas, offered art therapy as part of their psychiatric services to returning World War II veterans.

By 1980, a job series was established to facilitate the hiring of art therapists nationwide. The "GS638 Series for Creative Art Therapists and Recreational Therapists." Today, art therapists are employed in VA hospitals throughout the United

States. They offer therapeutic services to military personnel and their families in hospitals, clinics, mental health programs, and private practice.

HOW DOES ART THERAPY HELP VETERANS WITH PTSD?

Art therapy helps veterans in a variety of ways. For returning military with mental health conditions, art therapy provides emotional relief by encouraging expression of feelings and concerns. Art making is observed to relieve depression and anxiety as well as to improve reality orientation.

Currently, art therapists and researchers are studying the value of art therapy in treating post-traumatic stress disorder (PTSD), a problem experienced by many combat veterans returning from the recent conflicts in the Middle East and those from previous wars.

For the returning military suffering from PTSD, art therapy is used to reduce debilitating symptoms, provide opportunity for expression and resolution of painful memories, and enhance stress reduction through art-based relaxation techniques and coping skills.

In particular, art therapy helps by:

- Reducing anxiety and mood disorders
- Reducing behaviors that interfere with emotional and cognitive functioning
- Externalizing, verbalizing, and resolving memories of traumatic events
- Reactivating positive emotions, self-worth, and self-esteem.

Some veterans highly recommend art therapy programs to all the returned veterans to help them cope and adjust to new environments and divert them from committing suicide, which is on the rise. Do you know that over twenty veterans commit suicide every single day? (See Resources List at the end of the book for additional articles.)

Do you know that over twenty veterans commit suicide every single day?

One morning I was listening to National Public Radio (NPR) talk radio. The report was about PTSD. One young veteran asked his mother, "Do you believe in an afterlife?" His mother replied, "Yes I believe in an afterlife, but what are you trying to tell me?" He replied, "I killed so many people that I think I am going to hell." Some veterans with PTSD also feel guilty because they survived and their friends did not. It is called "survival guilt."

A reentry program with art therapy is highly recommended by many professionals and the veteran themselves. It works wonders, according to one Vietnam veteran. "You have to purge the sound, the smell, the feel in your fingers; otherwise you grit your teeth and might end up exploding."

"I killed so many people that I think I am going to hell."

According to some veterans, "There are so many good men and women returning from Iraq and Afghanistan that need to get the poison out, clean the wounds of wars. It will help them talk about and purge the gruesome events so that they can heal. The faster they get to art therapy treatment, the fewer problems there are down the road. And they need follow-up therapy too."

"You have to purge the sound, the smell, the feel in your fingers; otherwise you grit your teeth and might end up exploding."

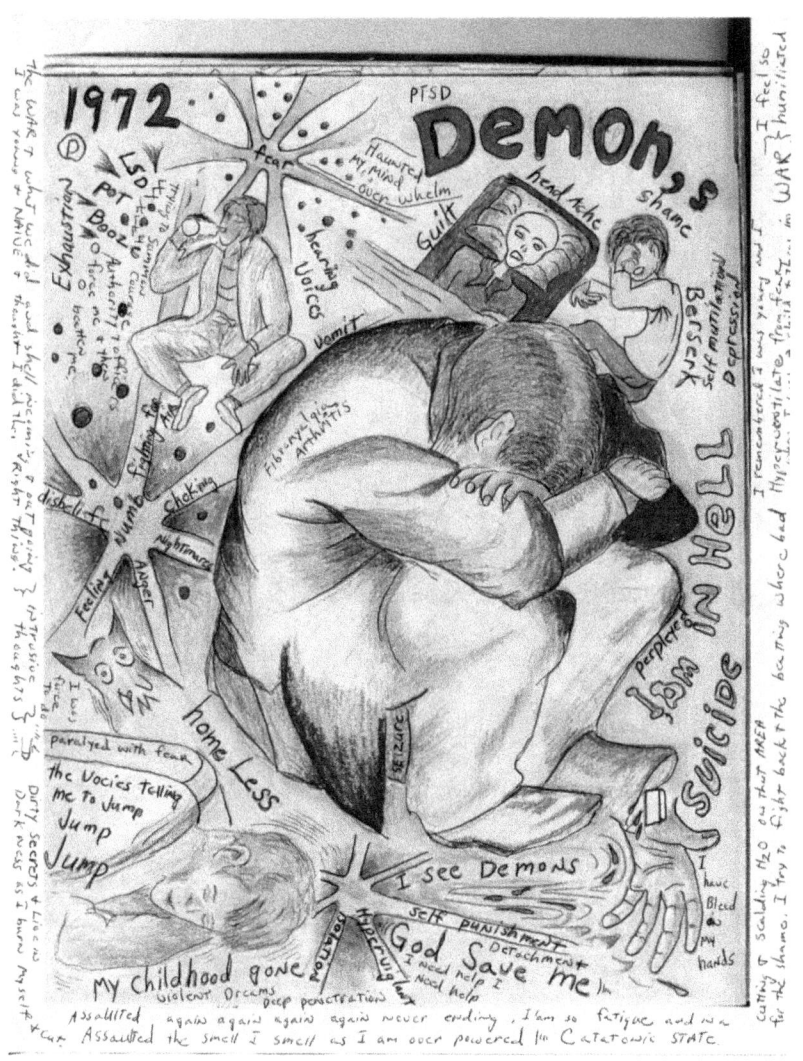

ART BY BIPOLAR DISORDER PATIENTS

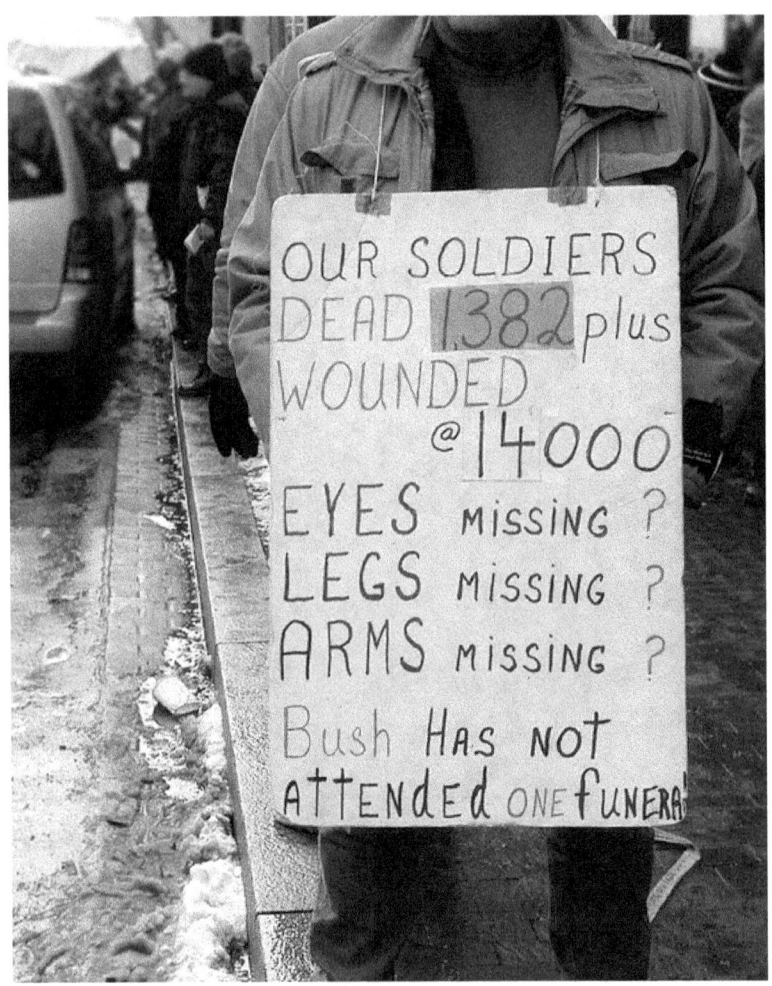

DISHEARTENED SOLDIER DISPLAYING THE HORRORS OF WAR

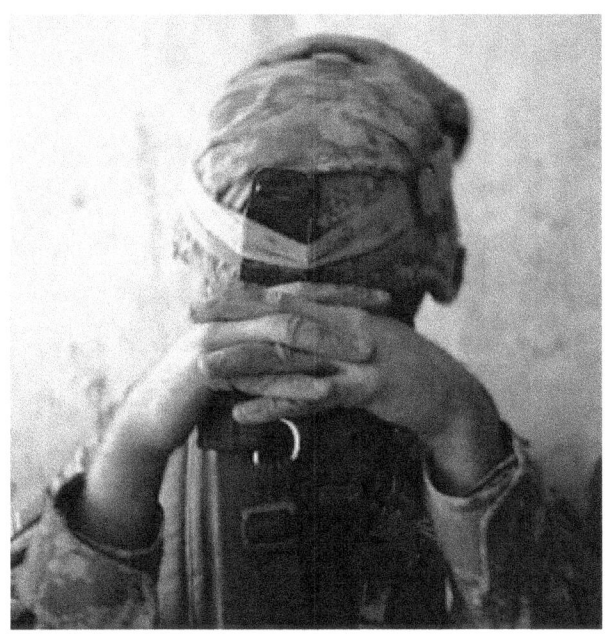

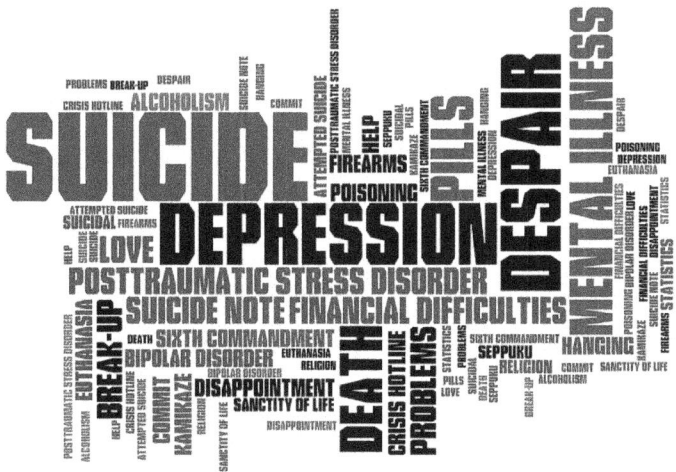

DEPRESSION

Depression can make everyday duties seem overwhelming. Taking responsibility for one's job or household responsibilities may feel draining. Many use medications to get past these feelings of apathy and tiredness. In many instances, talk therapy helps the depressed person hear for themselves what is going on in their heart or mind.

Quite often, learning how to recognize thought patterns and how to adjust them can be a significant part of beating the giant of depression. There is also another treatment, one that has been around for nearly fifty years, which also helps patients to combat depression through self-discovery.

Art therapy, like talk therapy, is a means of connecting with emotions, only instead of words, creative expression becomes the outlet. Art forms most often used by art therapists working with depressed patients include: painting, drawing, sculpting, dance drama, storytelling and music.

The ability to create something that is not yet criticized reveals inner feelings and is empowering. Group art therapy sessions tend to promote positive connections with other people, something that plays a key role in overcoming depression. When therapy is employed, patients find that art allows them to express thoughts and feelings that may actually be roadblocks to progress in traditional therapy sessions. This is because some emotions can be too painful to verbalize. Or, if the patient-therapist relationship is new, the telling of such hidden feelings may not feel quite safe. In either case, art allows a way for the person to give expression where words are not perceived to be an option. In this sense, art therapy is not intended to replace other traditional treatments, but works very well as a complement to other therapies.

Art therapy, like talk therapy, is a means of connecting with emotions, only instead of words, creative expression becomes the outlet.

In short, by creating a work of art, a person is given a means of externalizing powerful emotions that have been internalized. The person is left with a tangible form of what was an unspoken inner burden. Many patients report feeling as though just putting their feelings into clay or onto canvas has lifted an inner weight.

This may sound as though art therapy is only a means of expunging negative feelings, but that is only half of its benefit. Art therapy can actually be part of building positive feelings too. Tests have proven that creative expression releases dopamine, a chemical associated with the brain's pleasure or reward center. So dancing, painting, or playing an instrument stimulates the very chemicals which boost a person's feeling of well-being, reduces his/her anxiety and effectively works to combat depression. This is what depression medications are designed to do.

Art therapy was found to improve adherence to medical therapy and quality of life and was recommended as a component of therapy for heart disease.

However, patients looking to augment talk therapy or reduce the amount of medication they are taking may want to consider looking into art as a way to fight their current depression.

Art therapy may benefit patients with depression and anxiety commonly associated with heart disease. One study at a local U.S. hospital was performed on twenty patients with advanced heart failure in which, ten patients received art therapy and ten received no therapy once a week for six weeks. Art therapy was found to improve adherence to medical therapy and quality of life and was recommended as a component of therapy for heart disease. Art therapy was also found to be of benefit to older adults with mild to moderate depression.

MIGRAINE HEADACHES

Migraine is a disease, and while it's often associated with migraine headaches, the pain of the headaches is just a symptom of the neurological disease. Various treatments for the disease exist, including nutrition changes and hypnosis. An additional therapeutic method using art not only as a method of therapy but also a means to describe the disease has become more common.

CAUSES OF MIGRAINE

Researchers suggest that migraines are caused in part by a drop in the serotonin level of the brain. Serotonin is a chemical that serves a multitude of functions in the body, including regulating sleep, feeling of wellness and blood vessel health, according to an article published by Bryn Mawr College. See Resources List for additional information. Too little serotonin triggers constriction of the blood vessels, causing pain. Doctors believe this plays a significant role in the onset of migraines and also explains in part why art has a therapeutic effect on migraine headaches.

STRESS AND MIGRAINE

According to Web MD, emotional stress is one of the most frequently cited triggers of migraine headaches. Creating art increases the serotonin levels, which reduce tension, according to SelfGrowth.com. Proper serotonin levels discourage blood vessel constriction, allowing a free flow of blood to the head and fewer opportunities for migraines to develop. Art coupled with other therapeutic techniques like guided imagery or meditation helps relieve the tension caused by emotional stress.

From my personal observation at the neurology clinic, when patients come to the office with severe migraines, they look so miserable and in pain. When they look at the artwork on the wall where I display some of my work, and the beautiful surroundings and listen to soothing music, they really feel much better because of the relaxing, tranquil surroundings.

Creating art increases the serotonin levels, which reduce tension, according to SelfGrowth.com.

We make sure not use air fresheners, aromas or even flowers with nice smells because it might irritate them or trigger worse pain. Patients start asking questions about the meaning of a certain painting and they get involved and distracted for a while from their pain until they see the doctor for medical help. A serene, creative environment really does help. It raises their serotonin level and in turn helps them cope with pain, at least temporarily. Some patients buy my artwork because it makes them feel good!

Patients start asking questions about the meaning of a certain painting and they get involved and distracted for a while from their pain until they see the doctor for medical help.

VISUAL DESCRIPTION OF MIGRAINES

Art also serves another function in the treatment of migraine headaches. According to the Bay Area Pain and Wellness Center, sufferers of chronic pain have often exhausted all the means available to them to express the pain they are feeling. This means of expression is called Migraine Art. It bypasses problems encountered by the patient if communication between the patient and doctor is limited for one reason or another.

Migraine Art expresses the sufferer's condition to others in ways that words alone cannot. For example, blurred vision, an important indicator of the onset of the headache, may be difficult for a patient to describe. So the process of art helps improve communication between the migraine sufferer, her family and her doctor.

MIGRAINE ART

The movement toward expressing a migraine through art has come so far that there are now Migraine Art contests and gallery showings. These shows enhance awareness of the condition among the general public and medical professionals who treat migraine sufferers, according to an article published by Free Library. See Resources List for additional information. By holding this kind of exhibition, doctors can cross-reference the symptoms of other migraine sufferers, which helps them identify commonalities. In fact, these shows provided the visual information that first identified the visual apparitions associated with classical migraines.

HISTORY OF MIGRAINE ART

While it may not provide much relief, migraine artists may take some solace in knowing that they stand in good company. Artists like Vincent Van Gogh, Claude Monet and George Seurat all suffered migraine headaches, according to the Migraine Awareness Group. Artist and photographer Michael John Colman had such severe migraines that he considered ending his life rather than living with the pain.

There are many resources/publications and sites for migraine sufferers to find relief in artistic expression, such as:

- "Making Art Out of Migraines" - Etsy Blog

- Art and Migraines: Researching the Relationship between Art Making and Pain Experience

- Web MD, Migraines and Headaches Health Center

- "The Art of Migraine," Migraine Art Slide Show, NYTimes.com, March 3, 2008

- "Healing Photo Art Show" in U.S. hospitals, HealingPhotoArt.org

- Publications on Migraine Art Migraine Aura Foundation

- MigraineResearchFoundation.org

- Migraine Art, a book by Podoll and Robinson, The Migraine Experience from Within, 2009.

I have found all of above mentioned sites or publications to be very useful and informative. There are also additional references available on the Resources List.

EXAMPLES OF MIGRAINE ART

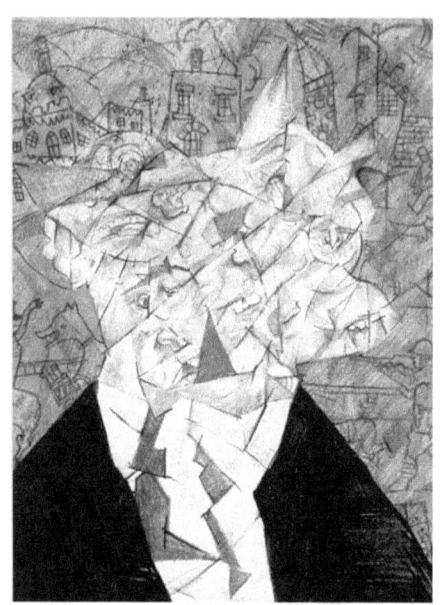

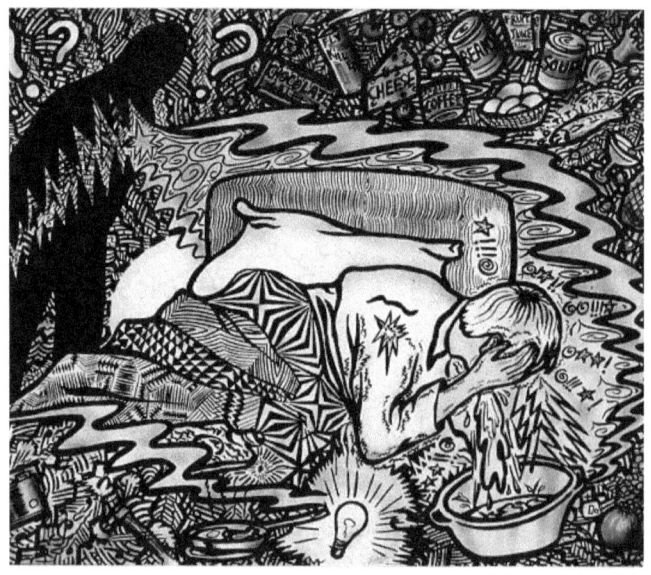

PHOTOS: COURTESY OF THE BRITISH MIGRAINE ASSOCIATION

EXAMPLES OF MIGRAINE ART

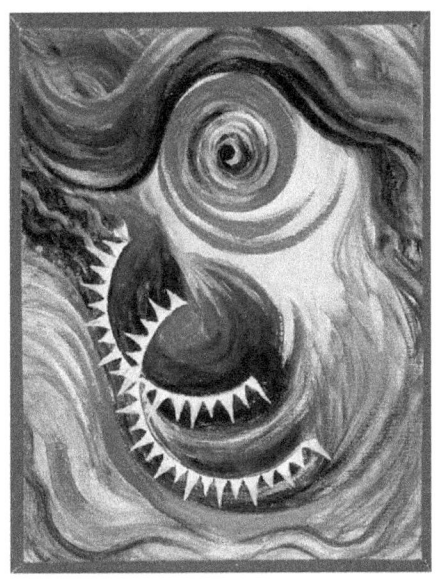

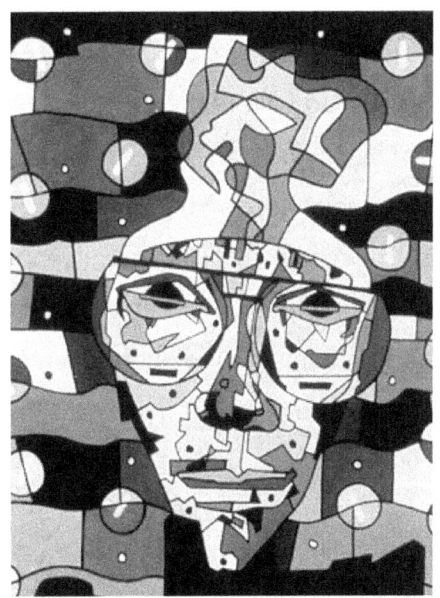

PHOTOS: COURTESY OF THE BRITISH MIGRAINE ASSOCIATION

FIBROMYALGIA SYNDROME (FMS)

Fibromyalgia (FM or FMS) is characterized by chronic widespread pain and a heightened painful response to pressure. Its' exact cause is unknown but is believed to involve psychological, genetic, neurobiological and environmental factors. Fibromyalgia symptoms are not restricted to pain, leading to the use of the alternative term fibromyalgia syndrome for the condition. Other symptoms include debilitating fatigue, sleep disturbances and joint pain. Fibromyalgia is frequently associated with stress, psychiatric conditions such as depression, and anxiety stress-related disorders such as PTSD.

Art therapy plays an important role in neutralizing symptoms associated with FMS. Art Therapy is a form of psychotherapy in which images in artwork are used in the same way as verbal communication in traditional psychotherapy. For a person with FMS or any chronic condition, verbal communication may fail to express what the patient is experiencing. In order to receive emotional/psychological support and learn to accept the disorder, the art therapist must connect with patient and understand the patient's status.

Typically, people with FMS who participate in Art Therapy, draw, paint or sculpt and then discuss what they have created. These discussions usually involve an art therapist or other people suffering from similar symptoms. A critical component of this discussion is a personal reflection and interpretation of the intended meaning behind the symbols or images that appear in the art work. Often, the images are more revealing and emotionally charged than verbal expression. It is a more direct, less threatening way of expressing thoughts and feelings than traditional therapy. The art creation process also helps to uncover unrecognized emotions and thoughts connected to FMS.

Art therapy plays an important role in neutralizing symptoms associated with FMS. Art Therapy is a form of psychotherapy in which images in artwork are used in the same way as verbal communication in traditional psychotherapy.

It is recommended that an FMS patient keep a visual journal throughout the art therapy program. The concept is similar to keeping a written journal, but it might contain drawings, paintings, sketches, photographs, self portraits, and other images that express unseen or unexpressed feelings or moods. FMS participants are free to explore any creative outlet such as wood working, stained glass art, song writing, weaving or any other creative method.

Art therapy is based on the belief that the act of engaging in creativity is healing by itself. For example, the practice of sketching how you currently experience your body will diminish the amount of pain your body is feeling. This is especially true for people suffering from FMS symptoms. There may be more or less emphasis on the meaning of images or on the underlying psychodynamics, depending on the patient's personal position.

Studies have demonstrated that creating art and engaging in the art process can change blood flow in the brain. Its' effect is similar to meditation. People often lose themselves in the creative process, forgetting about time and the demands of their bodies while working with art materials. People feel relaxed, refreshed, and stimulated during and after their creative process. Art therapy is highly effective in people dealing with overwhelming emotions or symptoms of pain, and especially effective for alleviating symptoms related to FMS.

For a person with FMS or any chronic condition, verbal communication may fail to express what the patient is experiencing. In order to receive emotional/psychological support and learn to accept the disorder, the art therapist must connect with patient and understand the patient's status.

EATING DISORDERS

Art therapy is a very valuable tool to treat individuals with eating disorders. Art therapists help patients move through the healing process using art, writing, music, gentle movement and guided imagery. Expressive therapy can also play an important role in addressing body image distortions and fear of body changes.

Body tracing is used as one particularly useful technique by art therapists to treat patients with eating disorders. Usually, the art therapist asks her clients to trace their bodies, and then to take a look at the tracing and explain and describe the figure. Then, the therapist has the client stand against the tracing and she actually traces their bodies. The results are shocking; the patient usually cannot see the similarities between the tracing and their actual figure because they are consumed with their own perception of their bodies.

Sometimes the therapist asks the patient to choose pictures from magazines, pictures of thin models, fashion models or movie stars, and asks them what they think about them and encourages them without judgment to express their feelings or their wishes to change certain parts of their bodies. This can teach them self-acceptance and to focus on the positive aspects of their bodies, to love their bodies and build their self-esteem. This technique provides rich opportunities to discuss their problems, perceptions about their bodies and to remind them that their bodies have more value in the world than just looking a certain way. Nurturing a true self-love for a body's abilities rather than perceived imperfections is a vital step towards living a physically and emotionally healthy lifestyle.

The patient usually cannot see the similarities between the tracing and their actual figure because they are consumed with their own perception of their bodies.

When I was going to art school in the eighties, there was one young artist in her late twenties. She was very thin and it seemed apparent to most of the students that she was not eating like the rest of us. One of my teachers was very big on emotions, feelings and self-perceptions, so once a month we used to have a session to talk about our history, experiences, trauma, problems etc. When it was her turn to speak, she was very nervous, embarrassed, and hesitant. Then she started talking, and she shared that she had an eating disorder and had no way to express the underlying wounds and trauma.

This technique provides rich opportunities to discuss their problems, perceptions about their bodies and to remind them that their bodies have more value in the world than just looking a certain way.

She continued to say that for some reason she had gravitated toward expressing her anger and confusion through art. So she used to pick up a pen and paper and scribble and scribble till she was exhausted and end up by breaking her pen and crumbling the papers. She kept saying she that had no choice, and that she was not in control of her body, and the only thing she could control was her eating habits. Then she revealed that she had been molested and abused at home, and so she felt all along she had no control over her own body and the only thing she could control was food. Needless to say, everyone in the classroom was in shock. Eventually, she went to an eating disorder clinic and underwent art therapy and talk therapy for a year. She made great progress in recovery and in understanding her wounds and tragedy. She said, "For the first time in so many years I was able to communicate verbally." She said that, for whatever reason, art led her to a new beginning.

OBSESSIVE COMPULSIVE DISORDER

Everyone double checks things sometimes. For example, you might double check to make sure the stove or iron is turned off before leaving the house. But people with Obsessive Compulsive Disorder (OCD) feel the need to check things repeatedly, or have certain thoughts or perform routines and rituals over and over. The thoughts and rituals associated with OCD cause distress and get in the way of daily life.

Celtic art therapy is very good to treat ADHD and OCD. Celtic art is ornamental, avoiding straight lines and only occasionally using symmetry. It is without the imitation of nature, but it includes a variety of styles and involves complex symbolism. There are three "traditions" of Celtic arts: Germanic, Mediterranean and British.

The style can be very complex and need concentration. It involves over and under interlacing, weaving, design and knots.

The Celtic art therapy provides rich opportunities to discuss their problems, perceptions about their bodies and to remind them that their bodies have more value in the world than just looking a certain way.

Individuals who have been diagnosed with attention deficit issues such as ADHD occasionally reject the benefit of a Celtic art therapy plate as being too involved for their mental state. This is likewise true of individuals who have been diagnosed with OCD. However, once introduced to the Celtic art therapy experience, these individuals are able to appreciate the passive state of relaxed awareness and often benefit from it.

Introduction of a Celtic art therapy plate to a person with OCD can be a very challenging task. The Celtic art plate is a very complex design that includes knots, continuous lines and very tedious and intricate designs that OCD individuals and sufferers of many other neurological disorders use in treatment sessions. The plate can be purchased from Amazon.com for $15-$35. The OCD patient is instructed to trace over the design slowly and calmly. It is critical to focus more on the "rules" for the Celtic art therapy experience. This supports an OCD individual's need for an activity's sense of logic and structure. Most often a "weaving" Celtic knot that crosses over and under presents a challenge for an individual showing her or his work. "Designs, such as the Celtic Trinity, the Celtic Wolf or the Celtic curls, work best with attention deficit and obsessive-compulsive disorder. Occasionally an individual with attention issues would be attracted to 'medium' or 'tight' designs, but this is usually not the norm. Individuals with OCD are rarely attracted to 'medium' or 'tight' designs, and can reject the entire Celtic art therapy experience when first exposed to anything but 'open' designs." For more information, go to www.celticarttherapy.com and see the Resources List at the end of the book.

The following is a specific observation made by Celtic artist Anne Raven's daughter with regards to attention deficit conditions:

A twenty-seven year-old woman with ADHD began to use the Celtic Trinity art therapy plate at the Michigan Renaissance Festival in 2010 where Anne was showing her work. The woman began to trace, but then began to talk excitedly while ignoring the plate. Anne guided to the woman to focus again, and again, and again-and after the fourth attempt at focusing, the woman finally gave her full attention to the Celtic art therapy plate. She traced the design for fifteen minutes without saying a word, and when she finally felt the desire to stop, she looked up slowly, blinked, and said, "My headache is gone". For more information, go to www.celticarttherapy.com and the Resources List at the end of the book.

EXAMPLES OF CELTIC ART

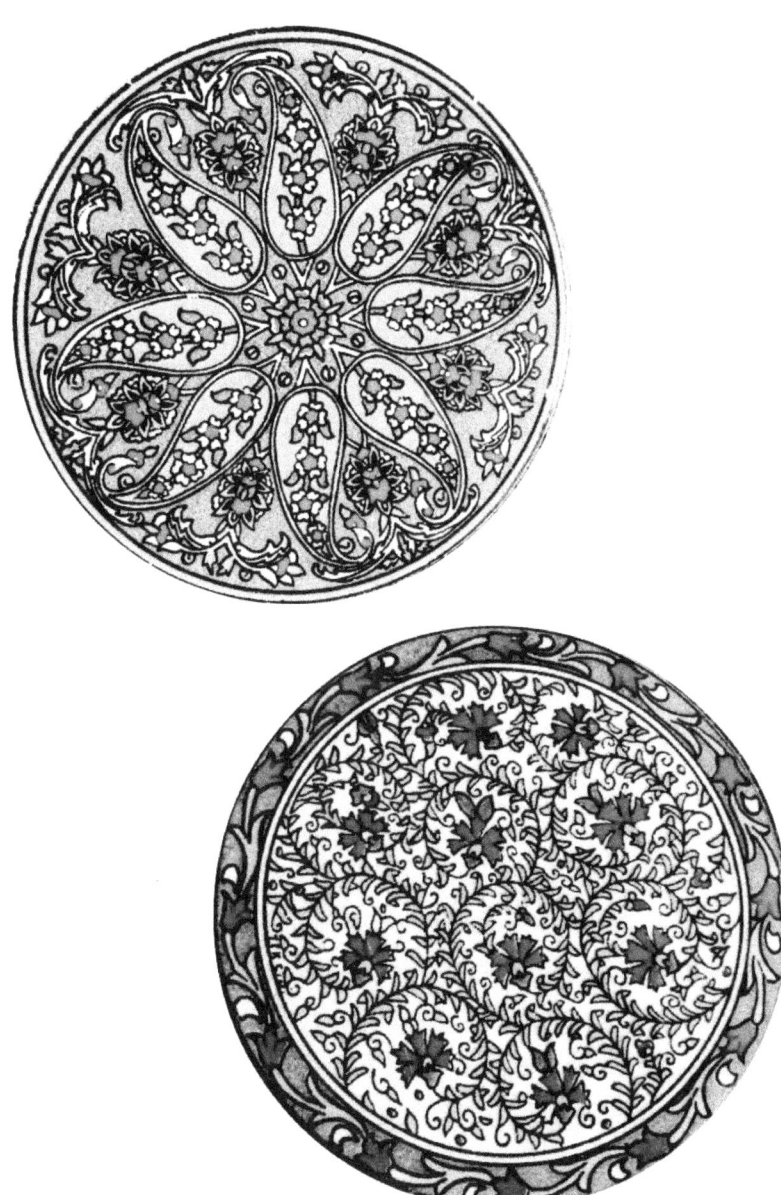

AUTISM

Autism is a neurological disorder that strikes children sometime during the first three years of life, affecting cognition, social interaction, and communication skills.

No specific cause for autism is known, but research suggests the disability might be genetic.

One of the hallmarks of autism spectrum disorders is difficulty with verbal and social communication. In some cases, people with autism are literally nonverbal: unable to use speech to communicate at all. In other cases, people with autism have a hard time processing language and turning it into smooth, easy conversation. People with autism may also have a tough time reading faces and body language. As a result, they may have difficulty telling a joke from a statement, or sarcasm from sincerity.

Meanwhile, many people with autism have an extraordinary ability to think visually - "in pictures." Many can turn that ability to good use in the processing of memories, recording images and visual information, and expressing ideas through drawing or other artistic media. Art is a form of expression that requires little or no verbal interaction. Art can open doors to communication.

Art is a form of expression that requires little or no verbal interaction. Art can open doors to communication.

All too often, it's assumed that a nonverbal person or a person with limited verbal capabilities is incompetent in other areas. As a result, people on the autism spectrum may not be exposed to the opportunity to use artistic media... Or the opportunities may be too challenging in other ways (in large class settings, for example). Art therapy offers an opportunity for therapists to work one-on-one with individuals on the autism spectrum to build a wide range of skills in a manner that may be more comfortable (and thus more effective) than spoken language.

The research is somewhat sketchy regarding the impact of art therapy on people with autism. The literature consists mainly of case studies and papers describing the observed impact of art therapy programs. Some of the papers written and presented on the subject, however, suggest that art therapy can do a great deal. In some cases it has opened up a whole world of opportunity to individuals with autism by showcasing significant artistic talent. In other cases it has created a unique opportunity for personal bonding.

Other possible outcomes include:

- Improved ability to imagine and think symbolically
- Improved ability to recognize and respond to facial expressions
- Improved ability to manage sensory issues (problems with stickiness, etc.)
- Improved fine motor skills

Please see the Resources List for additional information and articles.

EPILEPSY

Epilepsy is a neurological condition that affects several million Americans. Unfortunately, most people with epilepsy face discrimination and are misunderstood.

Many people living with epilepsy have not received proper medical treatment. Others face prejudicial stigma and discrimination due to their condition.

In my personal observations of patients living with epilepsy I have found that these patients have remarkable abilities to express their inner feeling from anger, joy, sadness and beauty. Art therapy and creativity allows people with epilepsy to reclaim and feel a moment in their life that they have lost during a seizure. Observations of art work created by patients with epilepsy reflect a wide range of beautiful colors, shapes and textures.

A wide range of impressive artwork created by artists living with epilepsy is displayed on Epilepsy.com "Studio E" is another amazing space that encourages and supports artists with epilepsy to take advantage of the art therapy program can be found at https://www.epilepsyfoundation.org/studioe.

All of the artwork featured at Studio E is available for purchase with proceeds benefitting the Epilepsy Foundation.

Some patients with epilepsy who have completed the art therapy program, cite art therapy as an amazing experience which has connected them to others suffering from the same condition.

Art therapy and creativity allows people with epilepsy to reclaim and feel a moment in their life that they have lost during a seizure.

Group art activities give patients a sense that they are not alone. Group art sessions promote feelings of confidence, support and self-accomplishment. The art process engages participants with a variety of sensory- rich art materials and enjoyable methods for the discovery of each person's unique capacity for problem solving and self- expression. Also, public sharing of artwork within a group exhibit is very exciting and validating for participants. Art viewers are exposed to a different perspective of epilepsy which increases awareness and negates the stigmas and prejudices associated with the condition.

Some patients with epilepsy who have completed the art therapy program, cite art therapy as an amazing experience which has connected them to others suffering from the same condition.

ART BY EPILEPTIC PATIENTS

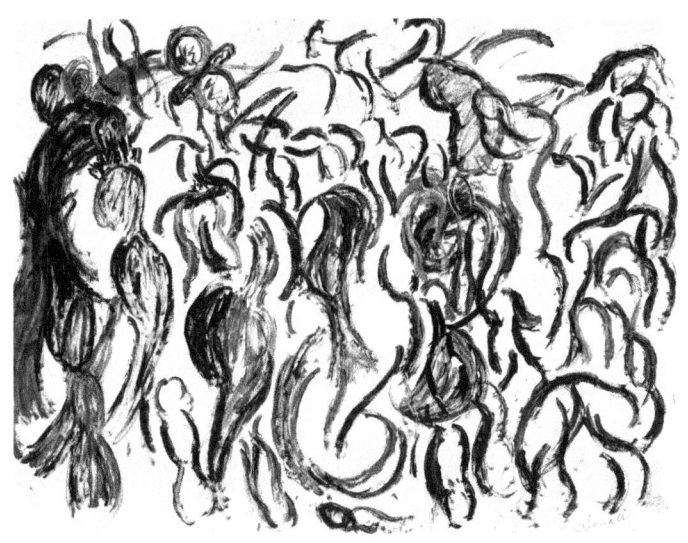

EXAMPLES OF EPILEPTIC ART

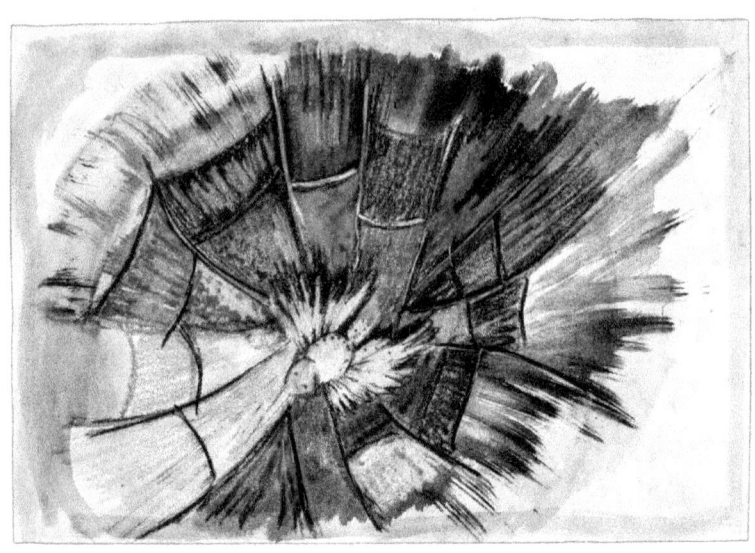

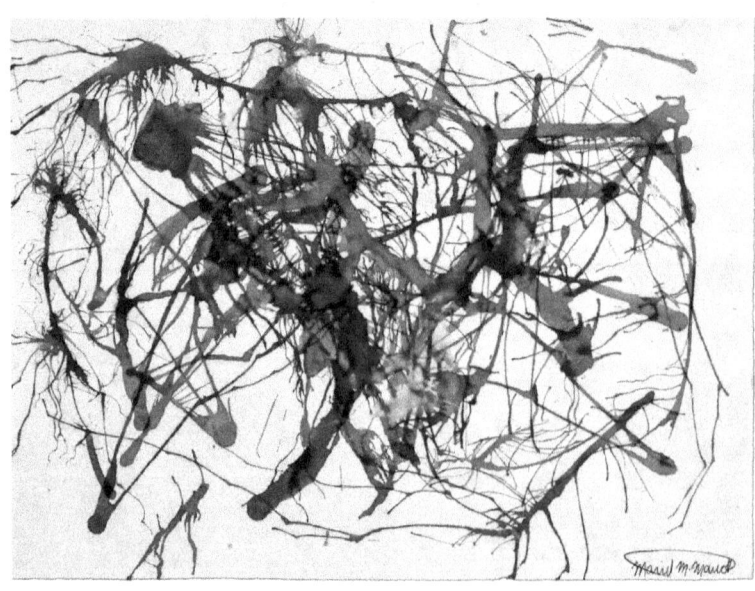

PAINT YOUR
STRESS AWAY

AMYOTROPHIC LATERAL SCLEROSIS

ALS, or Lou Gehrig's disease as it is commonly known, as progressive neurodegenerative disease attacking the nerve cells in the brain and spinal cord that control voluntary muscle movement. Symptoms include loss of mobility in the legs and arms, loss of voice, difficulties with balance, shortness of breath and a large variety of deteriorating functions.

Because there is no known cure for ALS, the course of ALS cannot be reversed. ALS treatments mainly involve efforts to slow the progression of ALS symptoms and provide patients with more comfort and independence.

I have collected many personal observations and insight on patients diagnosed with ALS through my work at the clinic and through my personal life. I have also the opportunity witness the value of art therapy for ALS patients first hand.

My lifelong childhood friend Suad was diagnosed with ALS and quickly turned to art and music to alleviate her symptoms and express her free spirit and passion for life when her body could not. My friend Suad was a beautiful person with energetic and adventurous spirit. She was always full of vitality and youth and her smiles carried innocence, freedom and excitement. Even though it has been many years since

146

her passing, I can close my eyes and instantly remember her contagious smile, giggle, passion for music and dancing.

When I visited her in the later stages of her illness, she would ask me to turn on her favorite song. She was so happy just to shake her shoulders and try to dance even though the rest

She cherished her limited mobility in her hands and would write to me explaining that she was grateful that she could paint and distract herself from her depression.

of her body could not. In her late forties, she started to lose balance, lose weight, struggle for breath and mobility.

Finally, she lost her voice, but she could still use her hands, arms, and shoulders. She instinctively turned to art to express herself. My friend Suad faced a dreadful diagnosis but never gave up. She could not talk but she could write, draw and paint. She started painting and painting, always in a hurry to finish what she started. Suad painted small paintings and greeting cards. Her paintings were beautiful using gold and turquoise colors; she painted on slips of black paper. She painted landscapes, portraits, shrines flowers and nature and mailed me many of them.

Art therapy became her escape from a very difficult and

deteriorating illness. Art therapy became my own personal connection to my lifelong friend and helped me really understand her in ways that words could never reveal. She cherished her limited mobility in her hands and would write to me explaining that she was grateful that she could paint and distract herself from her depression. Her beautiful soul was revealed in the purest way through her art.

After a short time, Suad lost her ability to use her hands. However, she left a large volume of artwork for everyone to cherish and admire. I still have many of her pieces and I often bring them into my life to remember our friendship and our bond. The influence and therapeutic value of art in my friend's last years of life was unforgettable and life changing for us both, and gave her comfort and happiness, and a voice in a very difficult time.

Shortly thereafter, I received a telephone call from her daughter Zainab telling me that her mother had passed. I was watering my rose garden at the time I received the call, I felt

The influence and therapeutic value of art in my friend's last years of life was unforgettable and life changing for us both, and gave her comfort and happiness, and a voice in a very difficult time.

deep sorrow, wept, paused and I cut one rose and I held it to my nose because I knew that Suad loved to smell roses.

Other ALS patients used art therapy to document their illness and emotions during the progression of ALS. One artist is Margaret McCmant Alexander. She published an article "Run until tackled: ALS and Me and provides a detailed description of her diagnosis, feelings, symptoms and opinions of her illness. The article quickly turned into a running blog where she described her condition and also posts updates on the progression of her art. Her paintings focused heavily on self-portraits documenting the different stages of her illness and the various depths of her fears, pain and sorrow. Her work and thoughts can be found at: alsandme.blogspot.com

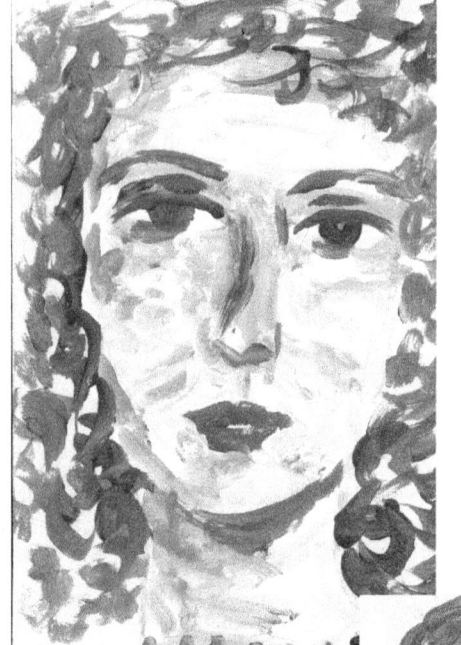

Portrait paintings by Suad of Ban (Hanaa's Daughter)

Portrait paintings by Suad of Hanaa

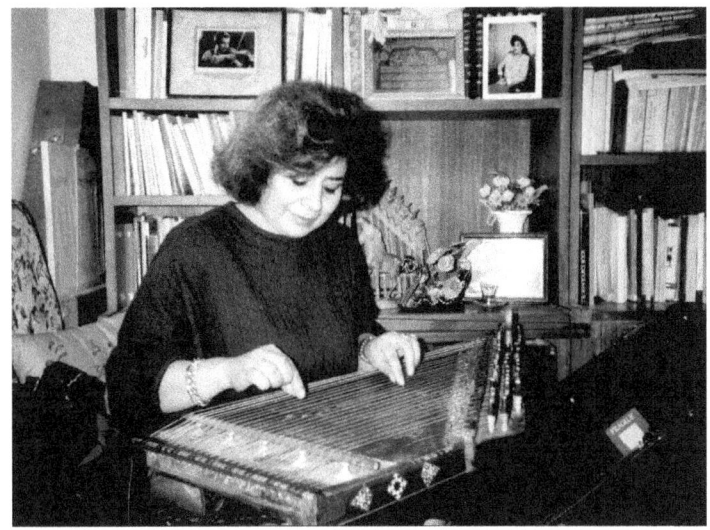

SUAD PLAYING THE QANOON INSTRUMENT.

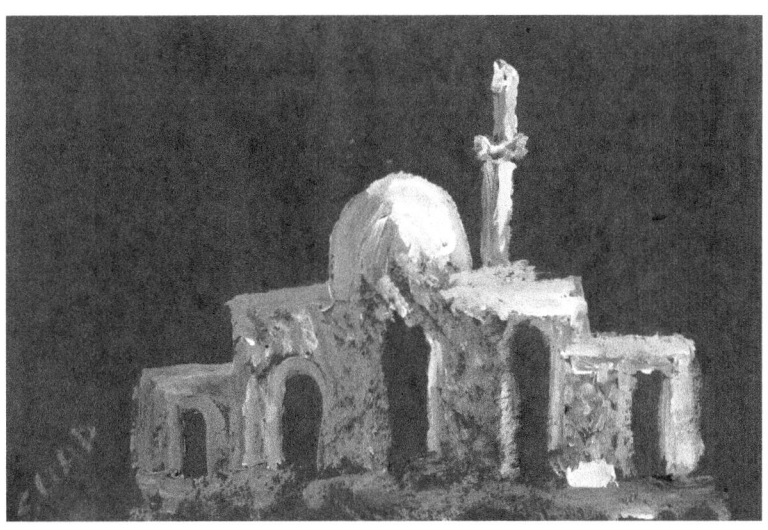

PAINTING BY SUAD OF MOSQUE IN BAGHDAD

151

PAINT YOUR
STRESS AWAY

CHAPTER 10

TAMING VIOLENCE
THROUGH
ART THERAPY

A rt therapy is commonly used in prison to reduce violence and rage among prison inmates. For example, in Pakistani prisons, prisoners learn to draw the intricate designs of carpets. Making these elaborate intricate designs is very tedious work, immersing inmates in the process. In return, inmates are calm, happy, feel self accomplished rather than bored, depressed and with nothing to do but contemplate harm and revenge when they leave prison.

Other art activities in Pakistani prisons include portrait drawing, crafts, and gift art making that actually becomes a source of income among the inmates. Sometimes the prison officials arrange for an art exhibit outside the prison to exhibit the inmates' work. The prisoners, after their release, usually never go back to prison and say that artwork gives them a

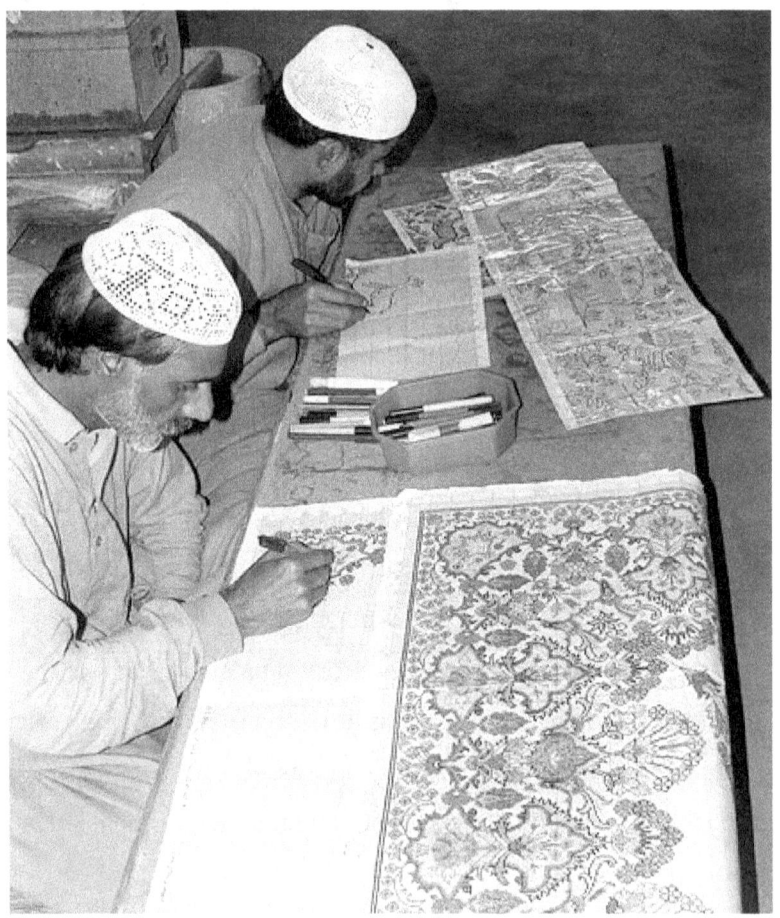

CONVICT ARTISTS BUSY DRAWING DESIGNS OF CARPETS ON GRAPH PAPERS

sense of accomplishment, confidence and sense of purpose. Further, they say the process has a magical effect on their psychology; it is very addictive, and they look forward to doing it again and again. See Resources List for additional information.

Prison officials say that involving the inmates in art therapy for long periods of time helps to tame anger, outrage, and hate and gives inmates a sense of purpose and confidence.

Art therapy is also used in Saudi Arabian prisons with inmates classified as terrorists. Prison officials say that involving the inmates in art therapy for long periods of time helps to tame anger, outrage, and hate and gives inmates a sense of purpose and confidence. Please see Resources List for additional information.

Also, art therapy has been used in Kingston prisons to help inmates access suppressed memories and emotions. Local therapist Sister K. Morrell often has clients draw landscape settings to illustrate how they see themselves. According to Morrell, artistic talent is unnecessary for art therapy. Artwork can have more than just aesthetic effects.

Art therapy is a form of psychotherapy that uses the creation of art to facilitate self-exploration and understanding. Participants use colors, shapes and imagery to express their feelings on subjects they can verbally articulate. Beth Merriam worked in the Kingston Prison for women as an art therapist from 1992 until the prison's closure in 2000. According to Merriam, in verbal therapy, an inmate's words would sometimes become jumbled as they spoke about experiences. "A lot of them were suffering from mental illnesses or they weren't receiving adequate treatment so they were unable to participate in verbal therapy," she said.

Art therapy is a form of psychotherapy that uses the creation of art to facilitate self-exploration and understanding.

While Merriam's services were sometimes requested, often the prison's nurses and psychologists would tell her which inmates would likely benefit from art therapy.

Her contract required her to work a few hours a week, but art therapy became more popular through word of mouth, so she worked up to twenty hours a week. Merriam said her job was initially overwhelming due to the wide range of personal conflicts among inmates, issues stemming from mental illnesses, sexual and substance abuse, self-injury and suicidal thoughts.

"Most women in the prison had experienced a lot of trauma and grief in their lifetime. It had piled up over the years so they had difficulty managing their emotions, so they would turn to using substance or other things to escape from society," she said.

Merriam was hired by Corrections Canada to work in the special needs unit after several prisoners committed suicide in prison. Working at the prison was Merriam's first job after graduating with her art therapy degree from the Toronto Art Therapy Institute, a private career college.

Merriam said art therapy allows individuals to reconnect with fear emotions in a safe way. She looks for themes in patient's artwork. "Art therapy can reveal issues associated with trauma, eating disorders and divorce," she said. "Art therapy allows patients to express their inner psyche on paper or canvas," Merriam said, adding that people of any age can use the practice for recreational purposes or self-healing.

"A lot of them had experienced a lot of anger" said Merriam, "and I think that many inmates were mothers and would draw happier times with their families. Even in drawing images of the outside world, there would be a window with bars." Painting, drawing and clay sculpture can all be used in art therapy, and patients actually choose what type of artwork that they would like to work on.

"Art therapy can reveal issues associated with trauma, eating disorders and divorce, Art therapy allows patients to express their inner psyche on paper or canvas,"

Merriam said something as simple as a patient's choice of tool can indicate their thought process. For instance, women with eating disorders often chose pencils, markers or other forms of the restrictive mediums to create the straight lines. This demonstrated a need for control, Merriam said.

"Over the years, I have observed a lot of it and it's not the symbols or images people draw, it's the way people go about art," she said, adding that someone with psychosis may create a disorganized piece.

Therapeutic value is found through informal conversation between an art therapist and patient as the patient creates a work, Merriam said. "Often in a conversation people share some of their thoughts…That is helpful therapeutically, so in a following session we will talk about the theme as they are working," she said, adding that oftentimes the theme would appear in the patient's creation. See Resources List for additional information.

PAINT
YOUR
STRESS
AWAY

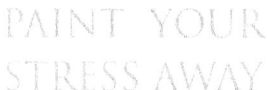

PAINT YOUR
STRESS AWAY

FINAL THOUGHTS

So you made it through. Congratulations! ***Paint Your Stress Away*** is a very serious and helpful book that can help you to manage your stress, tension, medical, physical and mental conditions. It shows you how to use art in your daily life or when you need it to solve problems and come up with solutions. You don't have to be an artist to use these tools, and you don't have to be a creative genius or have a degree in fine art to use them. You don't have to bother with the technical part; just concentrate on the process and the experience of doing it.

Taking the time and being serious about improving your health and immersing yourself and thoughts in the creative process to divert and cleanse your mind from your situation is the magic answer to lift your spirit and your psychological being. Art can even make you sleep better. When you do that, you will be pouring your stress, pain and tension all into the "art bucket."

I hope you read this book from cover to cover and watch the videos referenced in the Resources List to get the full effect. This book is easy to read book and filled with jewels of ideas and hints on how to improve your life and live stress free.

Hanaa F. Al-Wardi

PAINT YOUR
STRESS AWAY

RESOURCES

Internet address and telephone numbers given in this book were
accurate at the time it went to press.

A blinded pilot study of art work in a comprehensive epilepsy center
http.//www.ncbi.nlm.gov/pubmed/15710304

"ADHD and Art Therapy-YouTube"
http://www.YouTube.com/watch?v=n/OnVYJQuQE

"Agingmgmt.USC.edu"
Art therapy for Alzihmer's patients
www.arttherapyblog.com/seniors/art-activities

A Place For Mom
www.aplaceformom.com/...2013-8-3-art-therapy-dementia

"Art and Music Therapy for Alzheimer's disease"
www.webmd.com/alzhemiers/therapies-music-art more

"Art for the Mind, Body and Soul: ADHD and Art Therapy"
www.adhdarttherapy.org

"Art Therapy, PTSD and Veterans"
www.arttherapy.org/americanarttherapyassociation.com

"Art Therapy and Mindfulness Training Lower Stress in Breast Cancer Patients"
www.huffingtonpost.com/2110/12/02/art-mindfulness-stressrelief

Art Therapy: Art Therapy with Children and Adolescent ADHD

Art Therapy: Art Therapy Exercises for Depression

www.youtube.com/watch?v=n8z1bjdzanc

Art Therapy is helping Veterans combat PTSD/Fox4.com

Art Therapy

www.thefreelibrary.com

Art Therapy for ADHD and Anxious children

www.selfgrowth.com

"Beautiful Recitation"- Surratt al fajir-youtube

Calligraphy for Meditation and Philosophy Sutra "You are no body"

www.mumyouan.com/k/?T4026

Bryn Mawr College, Painting what we see with in

www.serendip.brynmawr.edu/biology

Calligraphy moving meditation workshop with Pearl Weng Liang Huang of Ru YI Studio

www.Youtube.com/watch? v=RY9rSKgcM51

"Celtic Art Therapy for ADHD and OCD"

www.celticarttherapy.com

Counseling and Support: Art Therapy at Memorial Sloan-Kettering Cancer Center

www.mskcc.org/cancer-care/counselin-support/art-therapy

Creative Sparks website, very important video on ABC TV station

www.artandepilepsy.com/art,epilepsy

Emotional Access through Art

www.queensjournal.ca

Guggenheim Study: "Art Education in Problem-Solving"

www.Learningthroughart.org/conference

Guided meditation-"The Seat"- YouTube

"Heart Sutra Meditation in Calligraphy" by Ponte Ryuurui YouTube

www.youtube.com/watch?v=QUVQYsaANTA

I Remember Better When I Paint

www.youtube.com/watch?v=54AtoQVGfwU

Uploaded by French Connection Film. Nov4, 2009

Margaret Naumburg Biography

www.goodtherapy.org/margaretnaumburgbiography

"Meditate with Calligraphy" by SW Anand KUI Bhushan-Youtube

Nov20, 2011-uploaded by Vedanta Klaude

www.youtube.com/watch?v=zzqoH7vlgM

Meditation Techniques: Short Guided Meditation for Anxiety

www.youtube.com/watch?v=ndlJ9fwhtYc

Oprah Winfrey, OWN network interview with Thick Nhat Hanh

www.youtube/watch?v=NJqUtWfs3U

"Pakistan: Behind Bars, Music and Art Frees Prisoners"
www.ipsnews.net/2010/11pakistan-behindbars-music-andart-free-
prisoners

"Saudi Arabia program to Rehab Prisoners": Crayons,
finger paint
www.creators.com

The Mindful Art of Thich Nhat Hanh-Calligraphic meditation
www.thichnhathanhcalligraphy.org

"The Sufi Whirling Dervishes of Istanbul"- YouTube
www.youtube.comwatch?v=whirlingdervishes.org

Using Art Therapy for Good Mental Health
www.maramcwilliams.com

Index

PAINT YOUR
STRESS AWAY